# Procedural Dentistry
## for
## *Complete Dentures*

# Procedural Dentistry for *Complete Dentures*

### Shivangi Gajwani Jain
MDS (Prosthodontics), Diplomat IBP(I)
Director, Academy of Dental Expertise (ADEx)
*Former Faculty*, Bharti Vidyapeeth Deemed University
Navi Mumbai, Maharashtra, India

*Foreword*
### Sandesh Mayekar

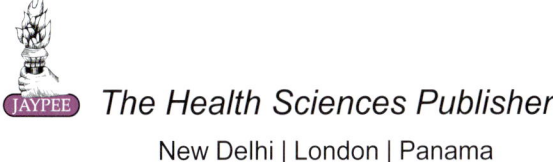

*The Health Sciences Publisher*
New Delhi | London | Panama

**Jaypee Brothers Medical Publishers (P) Ltd**

**Headquarters**

Jaypee Brothers Medical Publishers (P) Ltd
4838/24, Ansari Road, Daryaganj
New Delhi 110 002, India
Phone: +91-11-43574357
Fax: +91-11-43574314
Email: jaypee@jaypeebrothers.com

**Overseas Offices**

J.P. Medical Ltd
83 Victoria Street, London
SW1H 0HW (UK)
Phone: +44 20 3170 8910
Fax: +44 (0)20 3008 6180
Email: info@jpmedpub.com

Jaypee Brothers Medical Publishers (P) Ltd
17/1-B Babar Road, Block-B, Shaymali
Mohammadpur, Dhaka-1207
Bangladesh
Phone: +08801912003485
Email: jaypeedhaka@gmail.com

Jaypee-Highlights Medical Publishers Inc
City of Knowledge, Bld. 235, 2nd floor, Clayton
Panama City, Panama
Phone: +1 507-301-0496
Fax: +1 507-301-0499
Email: cservice@jphmedical.com

Jaypee Brothers Medical Publishers (P) Ltd
Bhotahity, Kathmandu, Nepal
Phone: +977-9741283608
Email: kathmandu@jaypeebrothers.com

Website: www.jaypeebrothers.com
Website: www.jaypeedigital.com

© 2017, Jaypee Brothers Medical Publishers

The views and opinions expressed in this book are solely those of the original contributor(s)/author(s) and do not necessarily represent those of editor(s) of the book.

All rights reserved. No part of this publication may be reproduced, stored or transmitted in any form or by any means, electronic, mechanical, photocopying, recording or otherwise, without the prior permission in writing of the publishers.

All brand names and product names used in this book are trade names, service marks, trademarks or registered trademarks of their respective owners. The publisher is not associated with any product or vendor mentioned in this book.

Medical knowledge and practice change constantly. This book is designed to provide accurate, authoritative information about the subject matter in question. However, readers are advised to check the most current information available on procedures included and check information from the manufacturer of each product to be administered, to verify the recommended dose, formula, method and duration of administration, adverse effects and contraindications. It is the responsibility of the practitioner to take all appropriate safety precautions. Neither the publisher nor the author(s)/editor(s) assume any liability for any injury and/or damage to persons or property arising from or related to use of material in this book.

This book is sold on the understanding that the publisher is not engaged in providing professional medical services. If such advice or services are required, the services of a competent medical professional should be sought.

Every effort has been made where necessary to contact holders of copyright to obtain permission to reproduce copyright material. If any have been inadvertently overlooked, the publisher will be pleased to make the necessary arrangements at the first opportunity.

**Inquiries for bulk sales may be solicited at:** jaypee@jaypeebrothers.com

*Procedural Dentistry for Complete Dentures*

First Edition: **2017**

ISBN: 978-93-5270-022-6

*Printed at: Samrat Offset Pvt. Ltd.*

**Dedicated to**

"Mom and Dad"

# Foreword

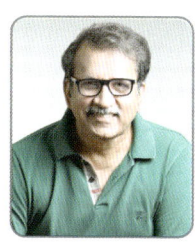

Dentistry in India has come a long way. Till the late eighties, dentistry was pain-related and was all about extractions, dentures, fillings, scaling and orthodontic treatment. After the introduction of Esthetic and Cosmetic Dentistry in the country in the year 1990, dentistry was looked at by people as something different from the past. The newer and higher technologies like lasers and the CAD/CAM in dentistry, implantology, composite laminate veneers, teeth whitening, temporomandibular joint (TMJ) and orofacial pain treatment and the advanced dental materials, equipments and techniques, a plethora of treatment options with predictable success has made dentistry glamorous. Today, people come to the dentists even without pain. Dentistry is constantly advancing and evolving by the day with the ever increasing demands from people to feel healthy and look better.

Around the world and in our country too, implants have become the norm for replacement of missing teeth. The entire implant procedure takes about 5/6 months, within which time, it is necessary to give the patient a complete denture, which takes care of chewing, speaking and esthetics. I personally believe removable complete dentures are very important as a first stage treatment option for replacement of missing teeth for many patients. If needed, these dentures can also be a perfect guide for the direction of the implant to achieve proper occlusion and aesthetics.

Education in dental colleges is based on curriculum recommended by the Dental Council of India. It consists of theory, practical and clinical knowledge backed by knowledge from reference books which is all fine and adequate to get through the exams. Most of the reference books contain the theoretical aspect of the subject in detail. However, the basics taught in dental colleges are the foundation to our careers in dental practice and cannot be ignored.

With regard to replacement of missing teeth in a subject like 'Prosthodontics', the students are trained to make complete and partial dentures. The learning process is under the guidance of teachers, and should they have any difficulty they can approach the teachers who guide them clinically and help the students to deliver the denture with proper functions like occlusion, phonetics, deglutition and aesthetics.

In private practice, if there is any difficulty in making a complete denture, a dentist needs a teacher as he cannot refer a college text book/reference books which are more into theoretical detail, so he needs books that acts like a teacher and can guide them to solve their problems. In short, a book that is in the form of pictorial, clinical steps, easy-to-understand and to the point is the best guide to a practicing clinical dentist and can be used as a "Reference Manual".

I am glad that Jaypee Publishers has come up with a practical and clinical oriented 'Procedural Dentistry book' that will be of great use to every dental practitioner. I am elated and happy that Dr Shivangi Gajwani Jain has authored the book *Procedural Dentistry for Complete Dentures*, the most important aspect of clinical dental practice.

The book is a perfect reference/Guideline manual that gives step-by-step procedures with techniques and newer materials, self-explanatory diagrams and clinically relevant pictures for all clinical situations. It is so beautifully written and presented in a simple, understandable way. Once you read it, every step feels easy. The book teaches you "how to do the best job".

I know Dr Shivangi as a prosthodontist and I have watched her very closely during her working stint in my dental clinic. She is a perfectionist, adheres to step-by-step procedures and adopts no short cuts, while ensuring patient comfort and satisfaction. She does not believe in "Chalta hai" attitude. This book penned by her is ample evidence of her exemplary qualities as a dentist.

**Sandesh Mayekar** MDS
MS in TMD and Orofacial Pain (USA)
Founder President of the Indian Academy of Aesthetic and Cosmetic Dentistry

# Preface

With the advent of technology, better understanding of the subject and availability of newer materials, we have entered an era where treating edentulousness with a fixed prosthesis has become the norm. So, when a patient walks into the clinic for a conventional complete denture, this is his last resort-we are his last resort. Compromised soft and hard tissues, debilitating health condition or financial handicap may be his reason for choosing this treatment modality. Whatever may be the reason, these patients of an advanced age have come to us for restoring their function and esthetics. The prosthesis must be designed and fabricated with an emphasis on preserving what remains. Educating the patient about the prosthesis, the first oral feelings with them, denture maintenance and eventually helping them adjust are part of the complete denture treatment.

Dentures have been a significant part of our undergraduate training as well. This book intends to help revise the basics for practicing clinicians, learn and understand the fundamentals for dental students and to create awareness about newer materials and concepts to simplify the process of denture fabrication.

"The gives" of this book:

- Understanding that each patient is unique and the treatment plan needs to be customized to fulfill their needs.
- As no two patients are same, the techniques and materials used to fabricate the complete dentures will vary and the clinician must be aware of the same.
- The transition from partially dentulous to completely edentulous is difficult and should be made in a systematic and coordinated manner.
- Why, which, when and how to use materials (new and time tested) to fabricate a functionally and esthetically successful complete denture prosthesis in a fast, predictable way.
- Recognizing that the preservation of oral structures is the only way forward.
- Understanding the psychological impact and role of treatment modalities such as immediate dentures, reline, repair and copy dentures.

Shivangi Gajwani Jain

# Acknowledgments

"To my Teachers and Patients"

It is with great pleasure that I take this opportunity to express my sincere and heartfelt gratitude to my friend Professor (Dr) Priya Verma for her constant guidance in the making of *Procedural Dentistry for Complete Dentures*. Without whom I could not have accomplished the task of writing this book. Her dedication, encouragement and suggestions have enhanced the quality of this book many folds. Thank you.

I thank Shri Jitendar P Vij (Group Chairman), Mr Ankit Vij (Group President), Ms Ritu Sharma, Director and the editorial staff of M/s Jaypee Brothers Medical Publishers (P) Ltd, New Delhi, India, who have given me a platform to bring in my creative ideas in to form of a book.

I am especially thankful to Dr Swati Mehra, Dr Harjeet Kaur Sekhon, Deep Kumar Dogra, Rajesh Ghurkundi, Arman Ali Idrisi and Vishwa Ranjan, of Jaypee Brothers Medical Publishers, for their hard work and unfailing support to give the correct shape, form and beauty to my book. To all those people who read, commented, assisted in editing, designing, proofreading, printing and helped in every small and big way to make this book a reality. To my publishers, Jaypee Brothers Medical Publishers (P) Ltd, who have given me a platform to write and present this book to a wide audience.

There are some friends and colleagues who have always been there for me, helping and cheering me on in all my endeavors. I am deeply indebted to Dr Gaurav Goel, my brother and friend and Dr Bijay Singh, Dr Snehal, who not only supported me throughout this process but also contributed few amazing pictures in this book. I would also like to thank Dr Snehal Jain and Dr Shilpa Dandekeri, for their contribution.

I am grateful to my Nanaji (Dr Kamal Kishore) and Nani (Smt Uma Rani), who look after me from heaven above. My Mom (Dr Madhu Gajwani) and Dad (Dr Rajesh Gajwani), for their unconditional love and unwavering faith, despite all my flaws. My father in law (Sri Ranjan Jain), who stood by me in every stage of completion of this book and my mother in law (Mrs Poonam Jain), who encouraged me to keep writing.

Astha, Rajat and Myrah, they fill my life with warmth and happiness. A special thanks to my husband, Prateek, without whom it would have been an impossible and lonely journey.

Finally, to God, who has always been generous and kind. Who has given me love for books, wild imagination, an unquenchable thirst to explore and an extreme sense of wonder. I feel blessed.

# Contents

1. **Anatomy Assessment** ........................................................... 3
2. **Preparation of Oral Cavity** ................................................ 25
3. **Impression Procedures for Dentures** .............................. 43
   - 3.1. Primary Impressions ................................................... 47
   - 3.2. Final Impressions ........................................................ 69
4. **Registration of Maxillo Mandibular Relations** ............. 87
5. **Anterior try in Aesthetic Considerations** ..................... 105
6. **Occlusion** ............................................................................ 121
7. **Laboratory Communication** ........................................... 135
8. **Denture Insertion** .............................................................. 141
9. **Denture Maintenance with Patient Education** ............ 161
10. **Special Techniques and Procedures** .............................. 177
    - 10.1. Immediate Dentures ................................................. 181
    - 10.2. Relining Procedures ................................................. 199
    - 10.3. Denture Repairs ........................................................ 211
    - 10.4. Copy Dentures .......................................................... 221

**Clinical Cases** ........................................................................... 233
- Case 1: Complete Dentures for Compromised Ridges ......... 235
- Case 2: Immediate Dentures with Chairside Soft Reline ..... 237
- Case 3: Denture Fabrication with Modified Neutral Zone Technique  241
- Case 4: Immediate Dentures ...................................................... 245
  - *Annexure* ................................................................................ 249
  - *Index* ...................................................................................... 253

# Step 1

## Anatomy Assessment

*"Nothing is more fundamental to treating patients than knowing the anatomy"*

*JP Okeson*

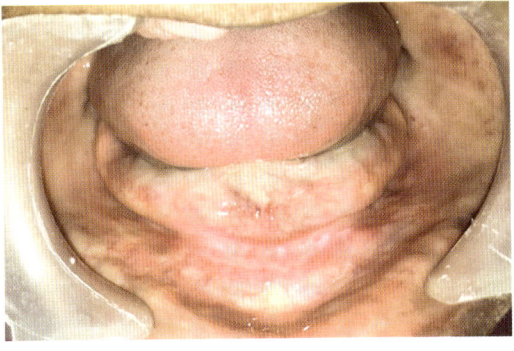

# Step 1

# Anatomy Assessment

## ■ INTRODUCTION

All patients who walk in our clinics are unique and so are their individual problems.

The anatomical changes due to extraction of teeth must not be studied in isolation. The physiological and psychological aspects of advanced age, trauma of losing natural teeth, systemic diseases, nutritional deficiencies and other related factors need to be considered while studying the anatomical variability. Though, for the fabrication of a successful complete denture prosthesis, the health of denture bearing areas is of prime importance. As a practitioner in today's era, we need to analyze all the clinical and patient related factors which may directly or indirectly affect the final outcome of treatment.

The alveolar bone loss is accelerated after tooth extraction. This causes various extraoral and intraoral changes. The rate of resorption is highest during the first six months of extraction of natural tooth resulting in a marked reduction in the width and height of the residual alveolar ridge. The remodeling of bone is a continuous physiological phenomenon, but the process is considered pathological when the rate of bone depletion is more than the bone formation like in periodontal disease, osteoporosis or trauma. Clinically, it is seen that the maxillary arch shows centripetal resorption, i.e. buccal aspect of the ridge is affected more, whereas the mandibular arch shows centrifugal resorption, i.e. excessive lingual ridge resorption eventually resulting in mismatched arches. Before starting the treatment, below mentioned examinations need to be undertaken.

## Extraoral Examination

- Temporomandibular joint (TMJ) examination **(Fig. 1.1)**
- Muscle tone
- Lip support **(Figs 1.2 and 1.3)**
- Facial form and profile.

## Intraoral Examination

- Denture bearing tissues:
  - Hard tissues: Residual alveolar ridge, supporting tissues and bony prominences
  - Soft tissues: Mucosa, lesions and freni.
- Saliva
- Tongue
- Examination of irreversible maxillofacial and oral lesions/pathologies.

## Radiographic Examination

- Orthopantomogram (OPG)
- Lateral cephalometric radiograph.

## Examination of the Old Dentures

- External assessment
- In situ.

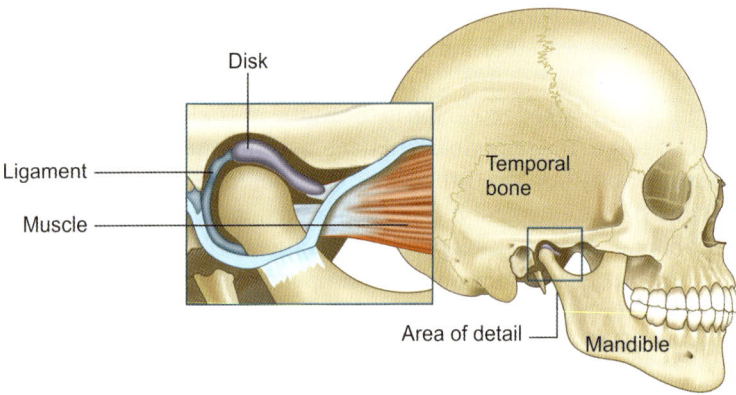

Fig. 1.1: Temporomandibular joint, condylar disc assembly inset

## Step 1 Anatomy Assessment

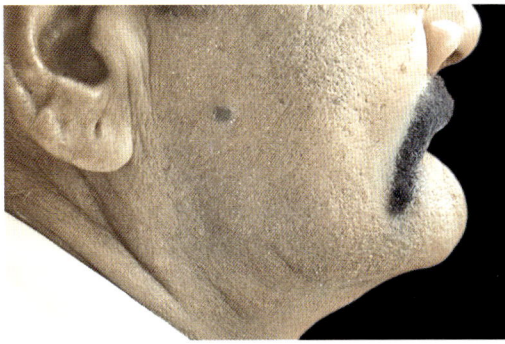

Fig. 1.2: Reduced lip support due to loss of teeth and alveolar ridge resorption

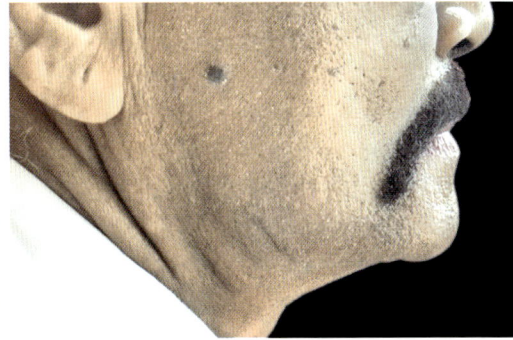

Fig. 1.3: Influence of complete dentures on lip support and soft tissue profile of the edentulous patient.

## ■ EXTRAORAL EXAMINATION

### Temporomandibular Joint Examination

A very common age related disease of the joints is osteoarthritis which even affects the TMJ, though comparatively less frequently than the other weight bearing joints. According to studies, 37 out of 100 adults have problems relating to the soft tissues that aid in the functioning of the joint efficiently.

Therefore, it is strongly advised to evaluate the joints for the following:
- Pain on palpation or on jaw movement
- Deviation of the mandible on mouth opening
- Trismus (reduced mouth opening)
- Unnatural sounds such as clicking.

These problems may cause difficulty in fabrication of the complete denture prosthesis. Hence, patients with such problems must be made aware of the limitations of the treatment.

## Muscle Tone

According to House, normal muscle tone with no degeneration is observed only in immediate denture patients. Most of our edentulous patients have slightly reduced muscle tone, while few may have greatly impaired muscle tone and function, usually accompanied with ill-fitting prosthesis, poor health, drooping commissures, exaggerated facial line angles and reduced vertical dimension (VD) leading to older appearance. Degree of muscle tension during rest or when stretched should be observed prior to denture fabrication **(Figs 1.4 and 1.5)**.

## Lip Support

Lips should be examined for cracking, angular cheilitis, candidasis, ulceration and fissures. The cause must be identified and removed before denture fabrication.

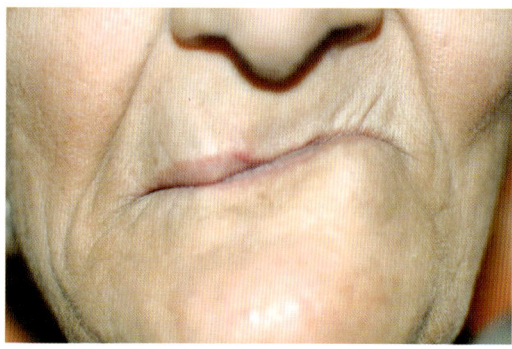

**Fig. 1.4:** Prominent chin with a class III profile and drooping commisssures

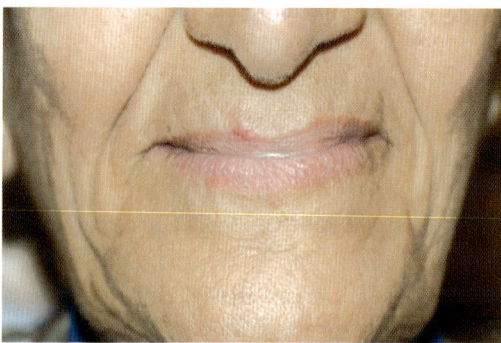

**Fig. 1.5:** A pleasing appearance restored with dentures in place

## Step 1 Anatomy Assessment

Lip support is an important factor which will directly affect the final appearance of the patient after denture insertion. It depends on various factors such as:

- **Lip Fullness:** Lip fullness affects the circumoral region by reducing excessive wrinkles, pushing out the lip commissures naturally and giving a more youthful appearance to the patient
- **Lip Thickness:** Lip thickness varies from patient to patient. A thin lip drapes around the artificial denture teeth, where in even the slightest labiolingual alteration affects the lip contour. Thus, changes the final appearance
- **Lip Length:** Studies prove that there is a direct relation between lip length and anterior tooth display. According to a study published in 1978, as lip length increases the amount of natural incisal display reduces **(Figs 1.6 and 1.7)**.. In some cases with excessive lip length, even zero incisal display has been observed **(Table 1.1)**.

Table 1.1: Lip length versus incisal display (JPD 1978)

| Lip Length | Incisal Display |
|---|---|
| 10-20 mm | 3-4 mm |
| 20-25 mm | 2 mm |
| 26-30 mm | 1 mm |
| 30 mm and above | 0 mm |

- **Residual alveolar ridge form:** After the loss of anterior teeth there is bone resorption causing loss of lip support which can be expressed as "falling in" of the lips and cheeks.

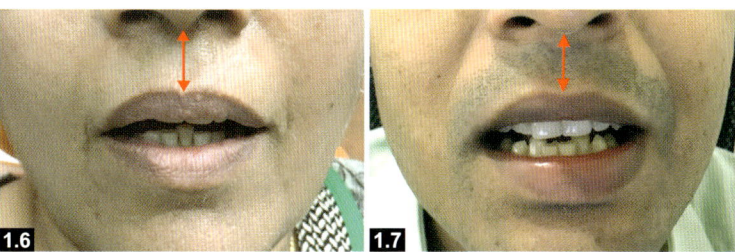

Figs 1.6 and 1.7: Lip length versus incisal display

Atwoods classification of postextraction changes in the adult mandible (1963) and Cawood and Howell's randomized cross-sectional study (1988) of changes in jaws, can be applied to understand the significance of ridge form on lip support **(Fig. 1.8), (Table 1.2)**\*.

The post extraction and knife edge ridge form are depicted in **Figures 1.9 and 1.10** respectively.

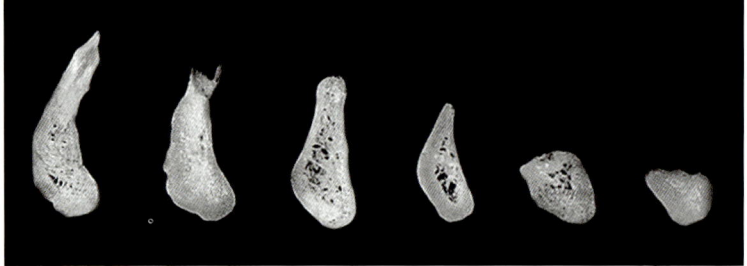

Fig. 1.8: Atwoods classification of post extraction changes

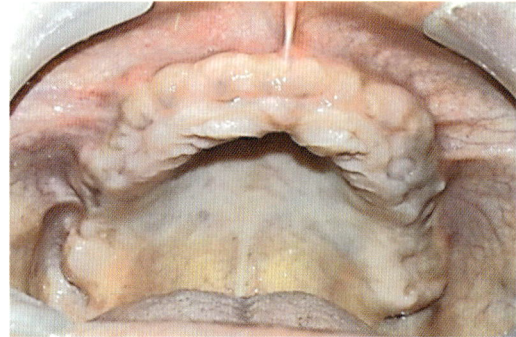

Fig. 1.9: Recent post extraction ridge. Uneven bony prominences can be seen as initial resorption is still in progress

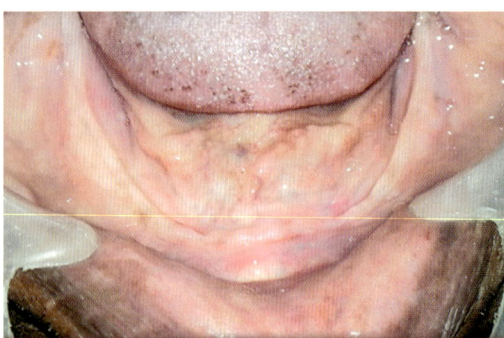

Fig. 1.10: Thin, knife edge alveolar ridge. Poor support for a mandibular complete denture

**Step 1** Anatomy Assessment

**Table 1.2:** Ridge form on lip support

| | |
|---|---|
| Pre-extraction (Well supported) | |
| Post-extraction (Partial lip support) | |
| High well rounded ridge (Partial lip support) | |
| Knife edge (Lip unsupported) | |
| Low well rounded ridge (Lip unsupported) | |
| Depressed (Lip unsupported) | |

\* Atwood DA. Postextraction changes in the adult mandible as illustrated by microradiographs of midsagittal sections and serial cephalometric roentgenograms. J Prosthet Dent. 1963;13:810-24.

## Facial Form and Profile

Many of the old denture wearers have reduced vertical dimension (VD) which can be assessed from the facial profile. The reduced VD makes the wrinkles prominent around the corners of the mouth, deepening facial lines **(Fig. 1.11)**.

Another consequence of collapsed vertical height is false mandibular prognathism, also called a pseudo Class III ridge relationship **(Fig. 1.12)**. The patient subconsciously pushes the mandible forward in an attempt to continue mastication with the worn out dentures. This results in approximation of nose and chin adversely affecting the function as well as the appearance of the denture wearers.

## ■ INTRAORAL EXAMINATION

### Hard Tissues

According to Winkler, "the size of the maxilla and mandible ultimately will determine the amount of basal seat available for the

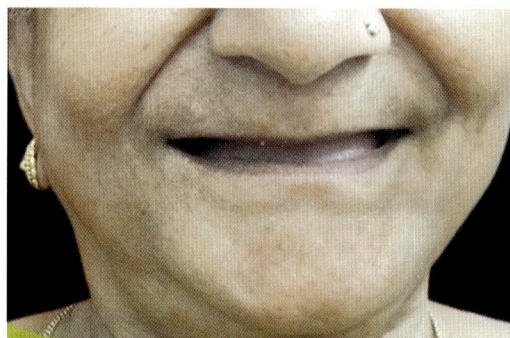

**Fig. 1.11:** Exaggerated line angles in edentulous patient

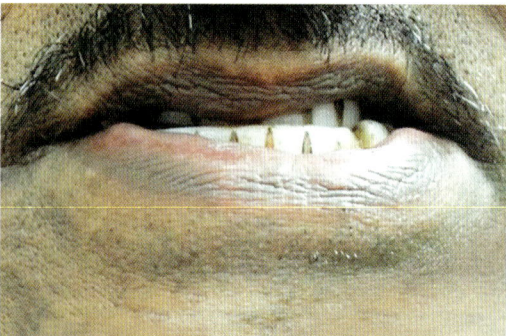

**Fig. 1.12:** An old denture wearer demonstrating a pseudo Class III ridge relationship with the mandible pushed in a forward position

denture foundation. Greater the size, more the support; larger the contact surface area, greater the retention. (**Fig. 1.13**).

## Height and Width of the Alveolar Ridge

Resorbed, shallow ridges are difficult to work on as important relief areas such as the incisive papilla, genial tubercle, mylohyoid ridge (sharp) and other anatomical structures become prominent (**Fig. 1.14**).

## Ridge Relation

Due to resorption patterns of the maxilla and mandible, many a times as practitioners we are faced with a smaller/narrower maxilla and a broader and larger mandible leading to a Class III positional ridge relation which gives the appearance of false prognathism.

## Hard Palate

Deep palates (**Fig. 1.15**) are difficult to record and the dentures are prone to fracture. Any movement of the denture base can cause loss of retention.

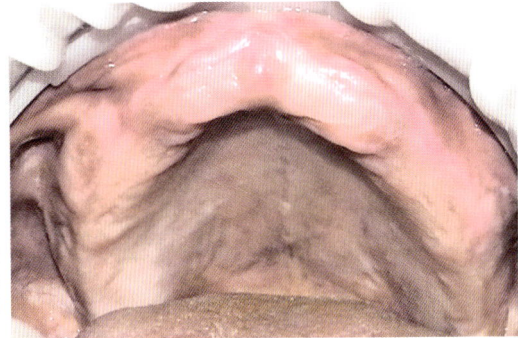

Fig. 1.13: A good size ridge providing more support, stability and increased retention

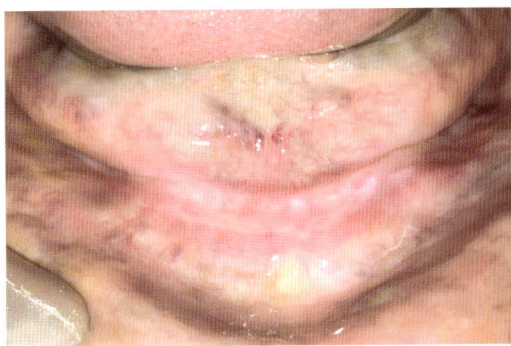

Fig. 1.14: Mandibular residual ridge with gross alveolar resorption

## Tori

Bony exostoses have an extremely thin lining of mucosa which if pressed by the denture will result in discomfort. Surgical excision may be required in large tori. Midline of the palate in maxilla and bilateral lingual tori **(Fig. 1.16)** in the mandible are common.

## Hard Tissue Undercuts and Presence of Spicules

- It is useful to note the presence of following undercuts for relief in the dentures:
  - Prominent mylohyoid ridge in the mandible
  - Undercut lateral to the maxillary tuberosity.
- Bony spicules if present in a wide area of the ridge must be smoothened by alveoloplasty before impression making. These areas if left unchecked, will result in pain and discomfort after final denture delivery.
- Small localized spicules if not removed surgically may be relieved in the denture itself.

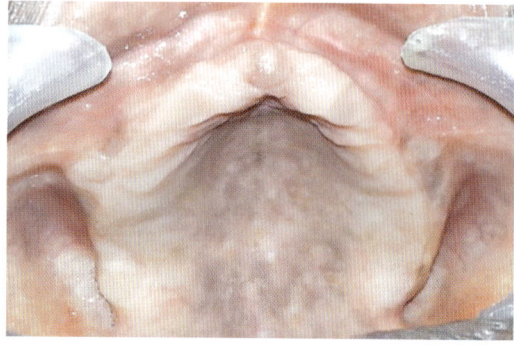

Fig. 1.15: Deep palates pose their own set of problems: Midline fractures, difficulty in recording the impression, loss of retention

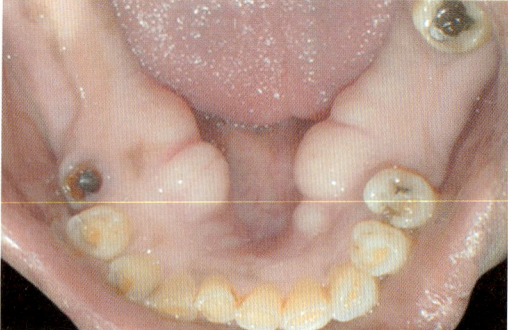

Fig. 1.16: Bilateral tori in the mandible: relief or surgical excision depending on the size and location of the tori

## Soft Tissues

### *Oral Mucosa*

- After a certain age in edentulous patients, mucosa shows signs of atrophy which varies in individuals depending on presence of systemic and localized health conditions. A healthy tissue is firm and resilient with thick mucous membrane
- Thin, atrophic mucosa is more prone to ulceration due to denture wear showing early signs of inflammation and discomfort to the patient whereas mobile, flabby, hyperplastic tissue causes denture instability leading to loss of retention **(Fig. 1.17)**
- The dentist must also look for common infections such as candidiasis as well as neoplastic changes/lesions in the mucosa.

### *Freni*

Presence and location of the freni along with vestibular depth must be noted and if needed altered (preprosthetic surgery) to ensure predictable complete denture fabrication **(Fig. 1.18)**.

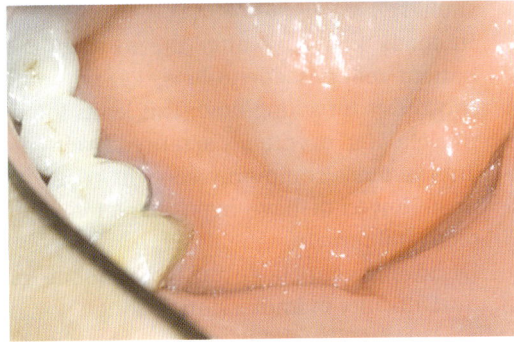

**Fig. 1.17:** Hyperplastic tissues: soft, movable, red inflamed tissues present in the maxillary arch

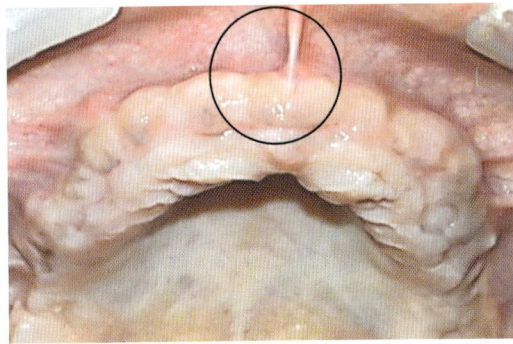

**Fig. 1.18:** Labial frenum: Location of high frenum attachments can lead to loss of retention

## Saliva

- The quality, i.e. mucous and serous content of saliva plays an important role in denture retention
- Excessively thick and ropy saliva may push the denture out compromising the stability of the prosthesis, while thin serous saliva creates an adequate retentive seal
- Saliva secretion varies in individuals. But, as the age advances, many patients develop conditions wherein they take medication daily for diseases such as diabetes, hypertension, and others. Many of these medicines affect saliva secretion and result in reduced salivary flow called xerostomia
- It is a problematic and fairly common symptom which affects denture retention resulting in inefficient mastication, speech and even denture sores. Diagnosis of such a condition is very important.

## Tongue

- The size of tongue is an important factor in mandibular denture stability
- In many instances after the extraction of natural teeth, the patient remains edentulous, i.e. without a complete denture prosthesis for a long time. This leads to relaxation of the tongue muscles and eventually acquired macroglossia/enlarged tongue
- This is most commonly seen in cases where the mandibular posterior teeth have been extracted and the anterior natural teeth still remain.
- Disadvantages of large and hypermobile tongue are as follows:
    - Difficulty in impression making
    - Denture instability
    - Tongue bite
    - Inefficiency in placing the food bolus on the teeth
    - Inadequate border seal due to shortened lingual flanges.

## Examination of Irreversible Oral Lesions

There are many reasons for the development of lesions/swellings in the oral cavity. According to an article published in the journal of cancer epidemiology (2012), oral cancer accounts for over 30% of all cancers in India with squamous cell carcinoma being the most common accounting for more than 90% of all cancers (oral oncology 2010).

## Step 1 Anatomy Assessment

As dentists, we are the first to observe these initial changes. Therefore, we are the first line of defense against malignant lesions which need to be diagnosed in their for the treatment to be effective.

## ■ RADIOGRAPHIC EXAMINATION

### Orthopantomogram

The purpose for analyzing the orthopantomogram is to screen jaws for presence of pathological/carcinomatous changes, impacted teeth, retained root pieces, unnatural radiopacities/radiolucencies and to analyze the amount of residual ridge resorption (**Figs 1.19 and 1.20**).

### Lateral Cephalometric Radiograph

Lateral cephalometric radiograph is used to assess the basic facial and dental proportions which may help in recording the correct VD at occlusion.

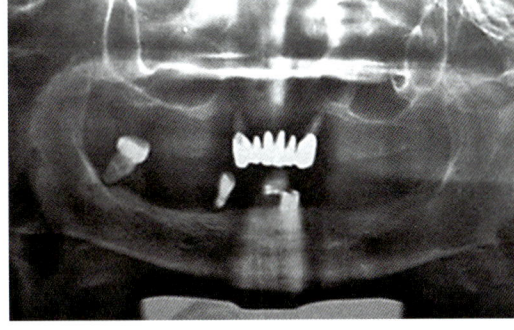

Fig. 1.19: OPG to be analyzed for screening jaws prior to complete denture fabrication

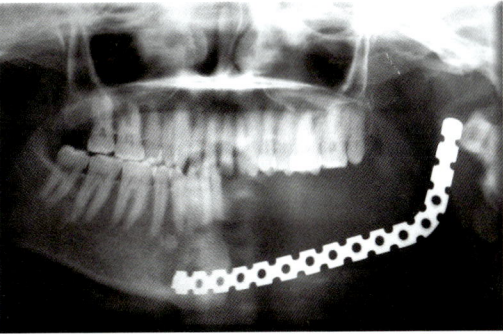

Fig. 1.20: OPG: A hemi mandibulectomy case, post surgical rehabilitation referred for a prosthesis

## EXISTING OLD DENTURE EXAMINATION

### External Assessment

The existing denture needs to be examined before construction of a new set of dentures for features such as:
- Fracture **(Fig. 1.21)**
- Repairs **(Fig. 1.22)**
- Signs of excessive abrasion **(Fig. 1.23)**

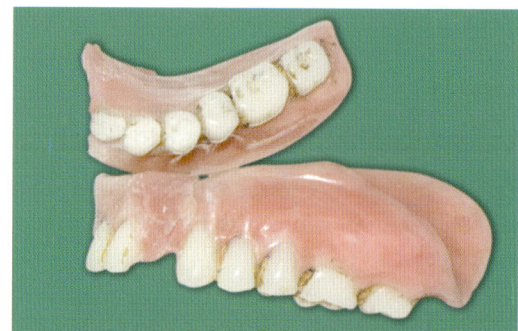

**Fig. 1.21:** Fracture of an old mandibular complete denture

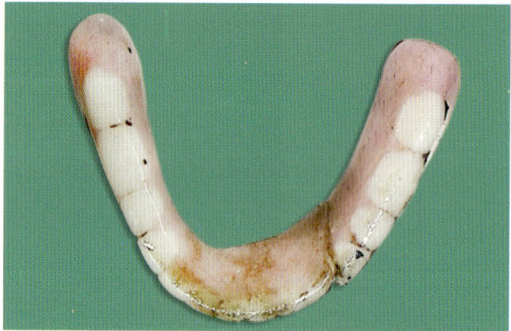

**Fig. 1.22:** Repair done by the patient using (at the counter) fixon resulting in mismatched denture pieces and immediate failure

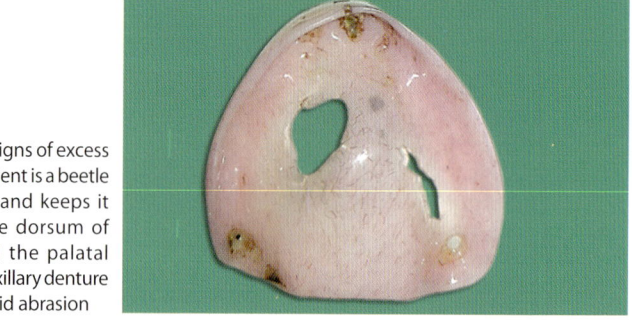

**Fig. 1.23:** Signs of excess abrasion. Patient is a beetle nut chewer and keeps it between the dorsum of tongue and the palatal aspect of maxillary denture leading to acid abrasion

## Step 1 Anatomy Assessment

- Abnormal wear and tear **(Fig. 1.24)**
- Stained dentures **(Fig. 1.25)**
- Washed out appearance
- Unclean and dirty looking dentures covered with food debris and plaque **(Fig. 1.26)**.

Problems in the old denture must be examined and dealt with, to ascertain that the same issues do not crop after the delivery of the new dentures. Fractures during denture wear most commonly occur

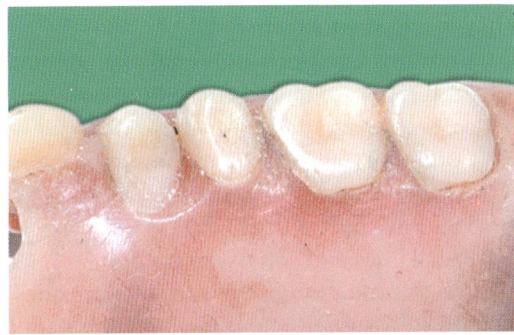

**Fig. 1.24:** Abnormal wear and tear of the denture teeth leading to loss in vertical dimension and forward shifting of the mandible

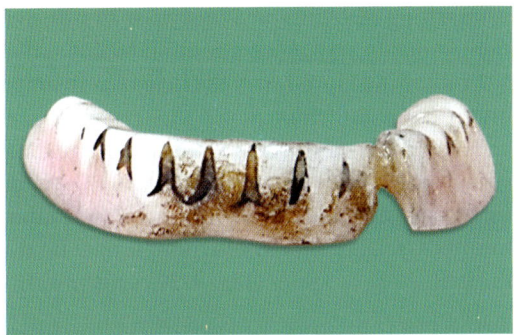

**Fig. 1.25:** Stained mandibular denture: Tobacco stains. History of chewing tobacco since 15years

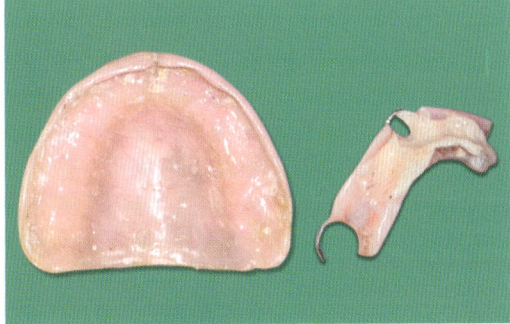

**Fig. 1.26:** Unclean and dirty looking dentures covered with food debris and plaque

at the mid line for maxilla due to flexion of the denture. Reasons, e.g. presence of mid palatine tori, deep palate, excessive labial freni relief, parafunctional habits such as bruxism/night grinding to presence of natural teeth opposing maxillary denture. Excessive abrasion or washed out appearance indicates incorrect denture cleaning technique. Stained dentures are common in smokers and areca nut chewers.

## In Situ Examination

Old dentures when placed in the patient's oral cavity must be checked for the following:
- Denture extensions and basal seat adaptation
- Posterior palatal seal (maxilla) placement and retromolar area coverage (mandible)
- Condition and position of the acrylic teeth
- Centric relation and maximum intercuspation
- Freeway space and VD
- Facial lines and soft tissue support.

The examination of the previous prosthesis in situ is extremely helpful in assessing the difficulties the patient faces with denture wear, along with the specific areas of denture construction where the dentist has to pay more attention to make the patient comfortable. VD can be measured with the help of a divider as two dots are placed on the nose and chin.

When the dentures are in place, applying gentle pressure will reveal the quality of adaptation. If the denture shifts/rocks with finger pressure then there is poor surface adaptation. If the denture bounces back or lifts in function, it may be over extended resulting in denture sore spots **(Fig. 1.27)** and instability whereas, areas of

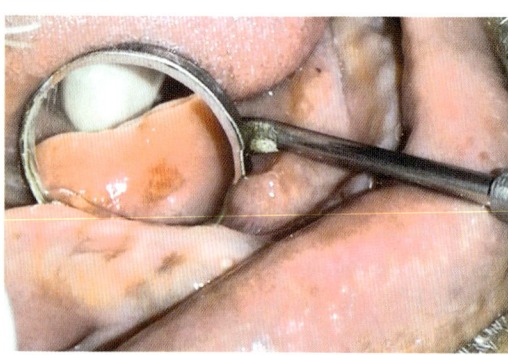

Fig. 1.27: Denture sore spot: seen as an inflamed reddish area on the lingual aspect of the mandibular ridge

under extension can be seen as space between denture border and vestibular sulcus. Commonly seen mistake is, that the mandibular denture does not cover the retromolar pad area where as the posterior palatal seal area of the denture is over extended. The anterior and posterior vibrating line should be marked in the oral cavity and transferred to the existing dentures to assess postdam.

Acrylic teeth get attrited after prolonged denture usage and may reveal the wear pattern of the patient. Probable cause of denture tooth wear are mentioned in **Table 1.3**.

Table 1.3: Probable cause of tooth wear

| Tooth Wear | Probable Cause |
| --- | --- |
| Excessive anterior tooth wear | • Improper patient bite<br>• Pseudo Class III<br>• Habitual centric positioning |
| Excessive posterior tooth wear | • Bruxism<br>• Heavy bite |
| Excessive over all tooth wear | • Night time denture wear<br>• Prolonged denture use<br>• Improper cleaning habits |

Ideally, patient's maximum intercuspation should coincide with the centric relation of the denture teeth but with old dentures it is usually not so. The slide, prematurities and any other discrepancy in denture occlusion should be noted.

The vertical dimension at occlusion and rest is evaluated and the freeway space is checked when the patient is wearing the old dentures. A reduced VD **(Fig. 1.28)** will show a marked deepening

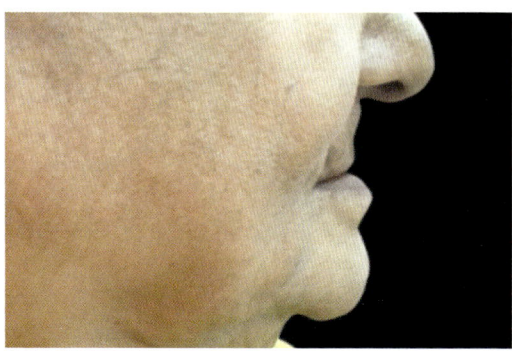

Fig. 1.28: Reduced vertical dimension: marked deep facial line unacceptable denture support. Biological age Vs Chronological age mismatch

of the facial lines, unacceptable soft tissue support and the patient will appear older. Most commonly, the over closure can be assessed by asking the patient to look forward and occlude. Then the patient is asked to relax and the VD is compared when the facial muscles are at rest.

After history taking, a thorough examination of the patient and the old dentures (if applicable), the clinician is ready to construct the new complete dentures. It is imperative that all the anatomical limitations and patient expectations should be discussed before starting the treatment to avoid un-achievable expectations leading to disappointment. **(Table 1.4)**.

Table 1.4: Examination chart for the clinician

| Extraoral | Normal | Pathological |
|---|---|---|
| TMJ | Normal | Clicking / deviation / pain / trismus |
| Muscle tone | Normal | Neuromuscular disorder / stroke / generalized loss of tone |
| Lip support | Normal | Deficient<br>Excessive / protruded |
| Facial line angles | Normal | Pronounced / deep / stretched |
| Facial profile | Normal | VD: Reduced<br>      Increased |
| Biological age versus chronological age of the patient | Normal | Enhanced |
| Intraoral:<br>Residual alveolar ridge | Well formed<br>Maxillary<br>Mandibular | Resorbed / knife edge / depressed<br>Maxillary<br>Mandibular |
| Tori | Absent | Present<br>Maxillary<br>Mandibular: Unilateral / bilateral |
| Mucous membrane biotype | Thick / normal / healthy | Thin / fragile / unhealthy / hyperplastic |
| Frenum | Normal<br>Maxillary<br>Mandibular | Labial, buccal, lingual:<br>High attachments:<br>Maxillary / mandibular<br>Low attachments:<br>Maxillary / mandibular |

*Contd...*

*Contd...*

| Extraoral | Normal | Pathological |
|---|---|---|
| Soft tissue lesions | Normal | Ulcers / Candida Infections / hyperplasia / redundant tissue / fibroma |
| Saliva (quantity and consistency) | Normal | Thick / thin<br>Serous / mucous<br>Dry mouth / excessive |
| Tongue | Normal | Enlarged / tongue tie |
| Surgeries / carcinomas | - | Hemi sections / radical / enucleation |
| X Rays:<br>Orthopantomogram (OPG) | Normal | Root pieces / lesions / impacted teeth / bony spicules |
| Lateral Cephalogram | Normal | Jaw relation:<br>Class I<br>Class II<br>Class III |
| Old dentures | Acceptable | Unacceptable |

## Conclusion

- After history taking, a thorough examination of the patient and the old dentures (if applicable), the clinician is ready to construct the new complete dentures.
- It is imperative that all the anatomical limitations and patient expectations should be discussed before starting the treatment. Good communication is the key to successful treatment and patient satisfaction.

# Step 2

## Preparation of Oral Cavity

*"Explanations before treatment are diagnostic,
those after treatment are excuses"*
*Charles M. Heartwell*

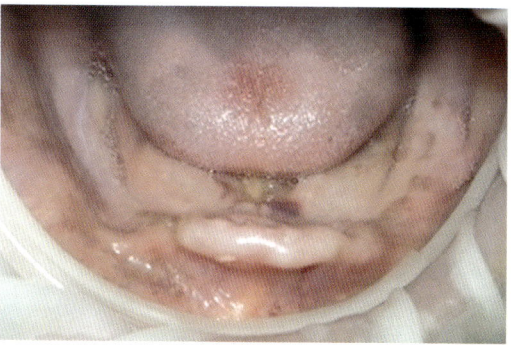

# Step 2

# Preparation of Oral Cavity

## INTRODUCTION

In recent times, humanity has seen a paradigm shift towards an increase in life expectancy of individuals due to improved medical support systems and newer medicines and procedures. Patients are likely to become edentulous fairly late in life. Any dental treatment specially a prosthesis like complete dentures which takes support from the underlying tissue needs to be analyzed and if required modified for it to be successful. Depending on the chronological age of the patient, psychological temperament and condition of the tissues the treatment plan varies.

After a detailed medical history and a thorough examination, the decision to make the changes in the oral cavity are made and the limitations of the treatment explained to the patient. If required, this is when another specialist may be included to correct or control existing systemic or localized disease. A pre prosthetic surgical correction should only be considered and executed once all non surgical alternatives have been evaluated. Preparing the Oral cavity for complete dentures is a process which takes time and effort on the part of the doctor as well as the patient. The difficulties needing tissue preparation can be categorized in three sections.

The problems depending on the time of extraction and the presence of old dentures are as listed below:
- Patients with terminal dentitions **(Fig. 2.1)**
    - Caries
    - Periodontal disease.

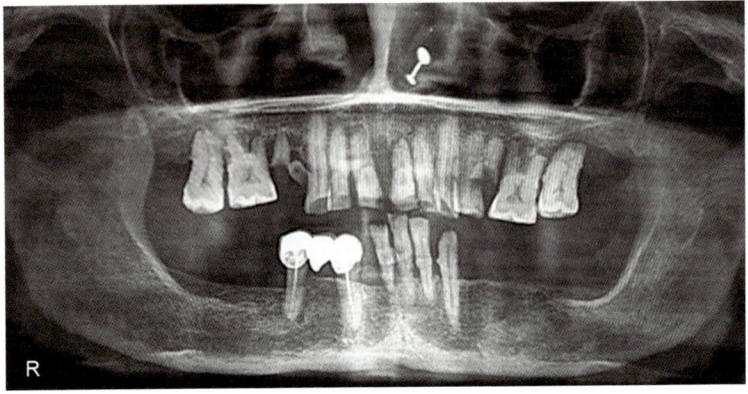

Fig. 2.1: Terminal dentition

- Edentulous patients, no past experience with Complete dentures ie: first time denture wearers
    - Retained roots and impacted teeth
    - Bony spicules or uneven inter septal bone
    - Hard tissue undercuts and tori/exostoses **(Fig. 2.2)**
    - Sharp residual ridge **(Fig. 2.3)**

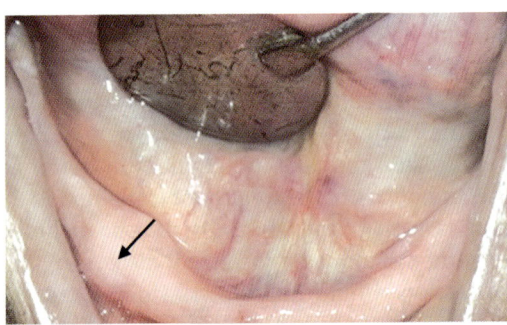

Fig. 2.2: Mandibular tori

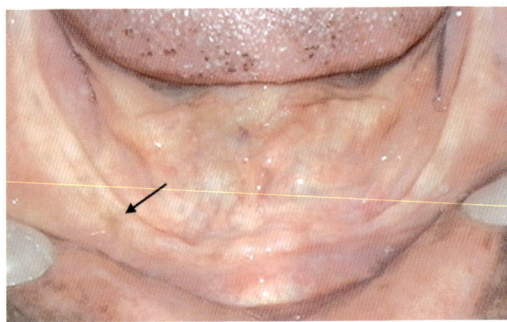

Fig. 2.3: Mandibular sharp residual ridge

**Step 2** Preparation of Oral Cavity

- ○ High and prominent frenum attachments **(Fig. 2.4)**
- ○ Low vestibular depth.
- Denture wearers ie: patients requiring a new set of dentures
  - ○ Soft hypermobile tissues over the ridge/flabby ridge **(Fig. 2.5)**
  - ○ Papillary hyperplasia **(Fig. 2.6)**
  - ○ Epulis fissuratum **(Fig. 2.7)**
  - ○ Denture sore spots

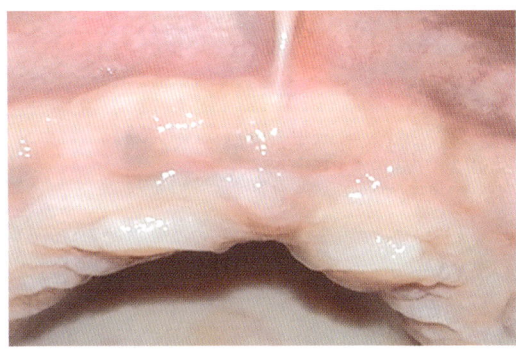

Fig. 2.4: High labial frenum attachment

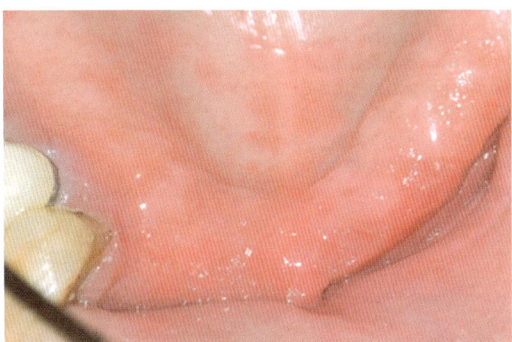

Fig. 2.5: Hypermobile inflamed tissues over the anterior ridge

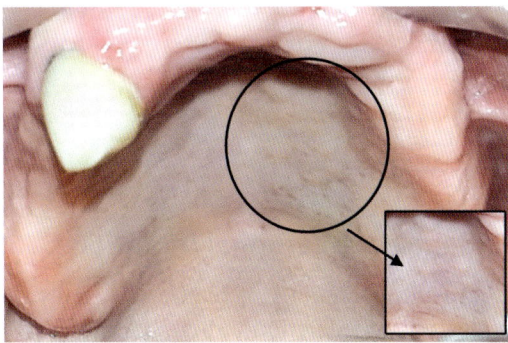

Fig. 2.6: Papillary hyperplasia

- Lesions: Candidiasis with angular chelitis **(Fig. 2.8)**
- Mucoceles and retention cysts **(Fig. 2.9)**
- Thin atrophic mucosa (compromised).

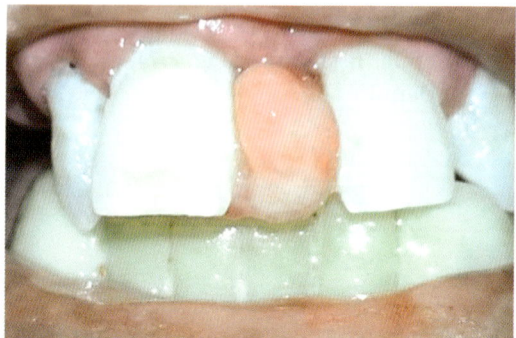

**Fig. 2.7:** Epulis related to an ill fitting partial denture facial view

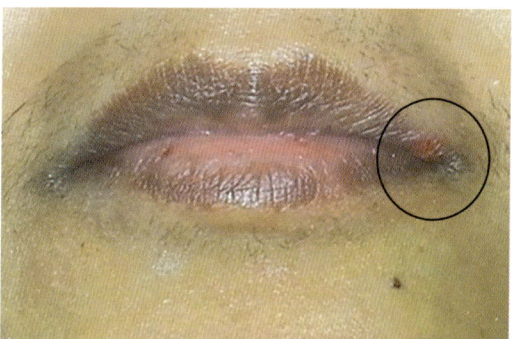

**Fig. 2.8:** Angular chelitis: Inflammatory condition commonly developed due to loss of vertical dimension leading to saliva dribbling in long term denture wearer

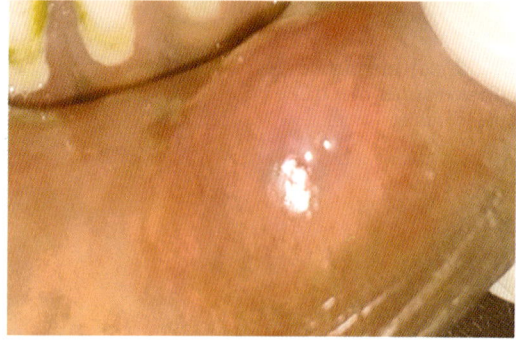

**Fig. 2.9:** Mucocele on lower lip: Caused due to localized trauma and obstruction of salivary duct

## Patients with Terminal Dentition

Complete extractions of teeth are usually done due to extensive caries, advanced periodontitis or pathological tooth wear (bruxism).

It is advisable to incorporate tissue corrections during tooth extraction, thereby negating the need for a second surgery.

In periodontally compromised situation it is best to limit bone reduction to a minimum as already there is phenomenal bone resorption.

## Bone Reduction

- Periodontally compromised cases:
    - Extraction
    - Rounding of sharp interseptal bone.
- Caries compromised cases:
    - Extraction
    - Alveoloplasty, undercut reduction.

# First Time Denture Wearers

## Retained Dentition

Retained roots and impacted teeth ideally should be removed before starting any prosthetic treatment, as they may erupt later. Many factors are taken into consideration before attempting surgical extraction of deeply seated teeth. Patient's general health and bone density being the most important. If the root/tooth removal will result in excessive bone loss, then an informed decision must be made to retain it. The implications explained to the patient and the tooth kept under observation for future changes.

## Hard Tissue Procedures

Procedure for removal of bony spicules, undercuts or surgical correction of unacceptable bony contours such as sharp residual ridge or exostoses is called alveoloplasty **(Fig. 2.10)**. This procedure is done by raising the mucoperiosteal flap to ensure adequate bone removal without excessive soft tissue injury. After smoothening the bone, the flap should be re-approximated and sutured. Depending on the extent of surgery, a surgical splint can be fabricated to help in healing.

## Hard Tissue Undercuts

Small undercuts do not necessitate their removal, neither the presence of unilateral undercuts. Undercuts that hamper the path of insertion of the complete denture prosthesis are:

- Bilateral posterior undercuts: Distal to tuberosity region
- Anterior prominent maxillary/mandibular ridge undercuts
- Undercut in relation to sharp and high mylohyoid ridge
- Combined anterior and posterior interferences
- In relation to tori/exostoses.

In presence of both anterior and posterior undercuts it is preferred to sacrifice bone in the posterior area as the preservation of anterior residual ridge takes precedence. The height and contour of the anterior ridge though being prone to increased ridge resorption is extremely important for denture stability. When the patient has bilateral undercuts distal to the maxillary tuberosity, one side is usually left intact whereas the opposite side undercut is removed.

Most common undercut in mandible is in relation to the mylohyoid ridge where the muscles attach. The superficial placement of this ridge and in cases with enhanced residual ridge

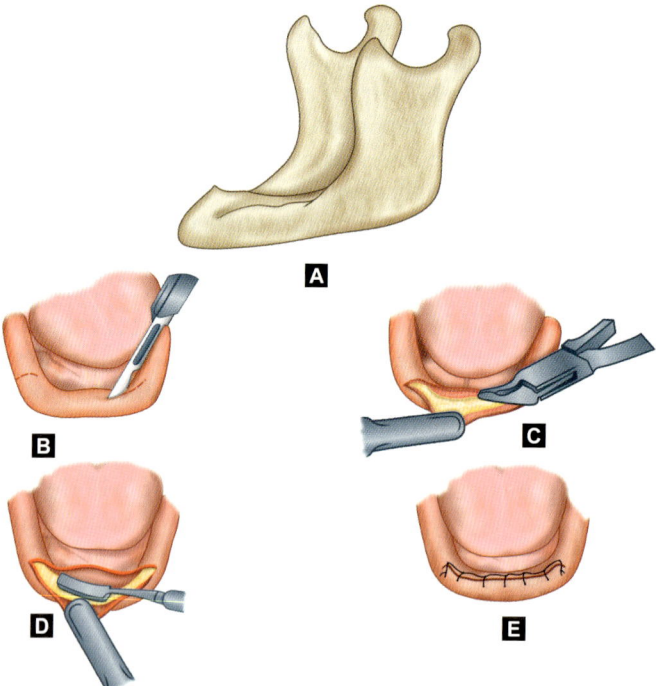

Fig. 2.10: Mandibular anterior ridge alveoplasty

resorption, mylohyoid ridge becomes more prominent interfering in denture placement and lingual border extensions. This ridge is surgically reduced only if there are chances of repeated ulceration/denture sores in the area.

In non surgical cases, the denture borders are kept slightly below the mylohyoid ridge and adequate relief is given in the area to ensure denture success without trauma to the tissues.

## *Tori*

Tori are benign bony prominences of unknown etiology. Commonly present in the middle of the hard palate in maxilla and bilateral mandibular tori in the lingual aspect of the mandible in vicinity of the premolar region **(Flowchart 2.1)**.

Thin mucous membrane stretching over the tori is usually prone to denture irritation. Small tori can be relieved in the denture but may be surgically reduced or removed if they act as a fulcrum or interfere with denture placement and stability.

Soft tissue anomalies can be easily corrected via minor oral surgeries, there by improving the foundation of the denture bearing area **(Fig. 2.11)**.

## *High Frenum Attachments*

The loose connective tissue attachments from the sulcus to the mucous membrane of the ridge, if encroach upon the denture bearing area can be removed or repositioned.

It is preferable to give enough space in the denture as frenal notches to accommodate the high frenum attachments going the non surgical way.

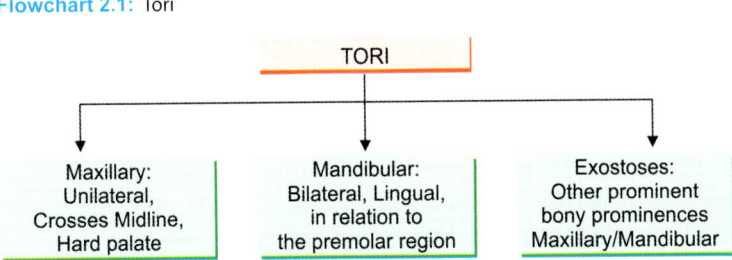

**Flowchart 2.1:** Tori

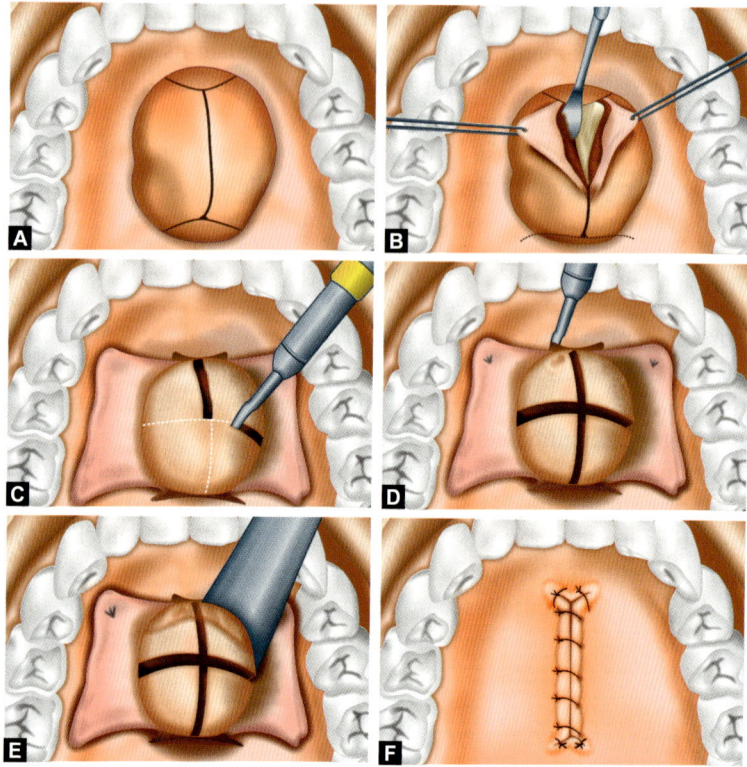

**Fig. 2.11:** Surgical removal of mid palatine torus

## Low Vestibular Depth

As mentioned earlier, a surgical intervention should only be carried out when all other means of accommodating the problem have been evaluated and found lacking. The surgical intervention may leave a scar thereby further compromising denture stability. Therefore, the doctor has to very careful during the surgery and should place a repositioning stent to maintain the new position until denture placement.

### Corrective Surgery

Vestibuloplasty is a procedure wherein the muscle attachments to ridge are lowered and the vestibular sulcus deepened. This results in increase in alveolar ridge height and better denture stability and support.

## Previous Denture Wearers: Common Features Of Abused Mucosa

### Soft Hypermobile Tissues Over the Ridge

Unstable soft tissues are usually found under poorly fitting old denture prosthesis. Ridge resorption which is a physiologic process turns pathologic due to unstable dentures resulting in excessive bone loss and redundant soft tissue formation on the ridge. This hyperplastic tissue formed due to malocclusion of old ill-fitting dentures further leads to denture instability and sores.

*Correction*

Small inflamed lesions may reduce in size once the denture is either left out of the oral cavity for a few days or with the help of tissue conditioners **(Fig. 2.12)**.

Large, fibrous, long standing lesions which do not resolve after conditioning and will get displaced during mastication are candidates for surgical correction. Sharp dissection with blade, electrosurgery or laser can be used for the same

### Papillary Hyperplasia

Multiple soft tissue projections commonly present on palatal vault, in relation to an ill-fitting maxillary denture combined with presence of mandibular anterior natural teeth. This leads to unequal occlusal forces and denture instability. Thus, the papillary projections are a result of poorly fitting dentures, localized long standing irritation coupled with mild oral infections such as candidiasis.

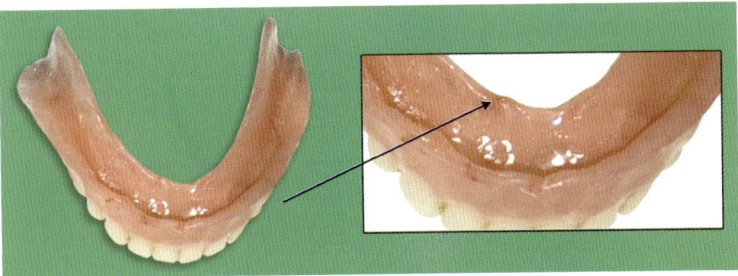

Fig. 2.12: Tissue conditioner placed on the intaglio surface of a mandibular complete denture prosthesis

*Correction*

Early hyperplastic lesions may resolve with tissue conditioning or keeping the denture out for a few days. Larger lesions may be surgically removed.

Similarly, epuli due to localized irritation in the flange region/sulcus are mostly reversible if the denture is either relieved or shortened in that particular area. Lining with Soft denture liners to condition the tissue also helps. Larger redundant tissues need surgical treatment.

## ■ SOFT TISSUE LESIONS IN DENTURE WEARERS

Treating any pathological lesion in the basal seat area is imperative as the presence of inflammation related to candida or lichen planus, angular chelitis or any such infection will lead to compromised retention and stability of the new dentures. Most common lesion is candidiasis and has various causative factors.

## Candidiasis

It is a fungal infection caused by *candida albicans*. The aeiotology of candidiasis is elaborated in **Figure 2.13**. The **Figure 2.14** shows a clinical presentation of infection.

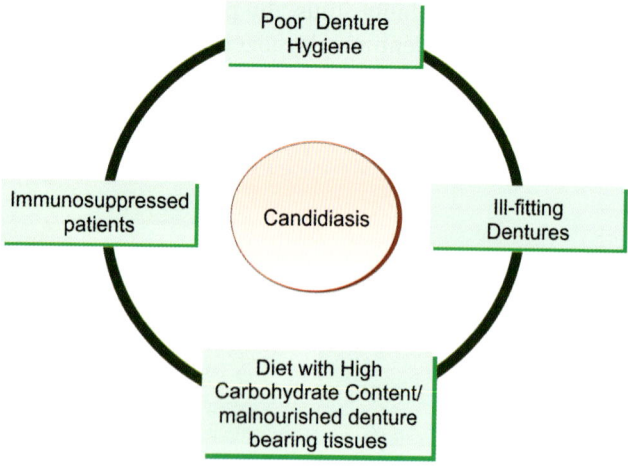

Fig. 2.13: Aetiology of candidiasis

## Step 2 Preparation of Oral Cavity

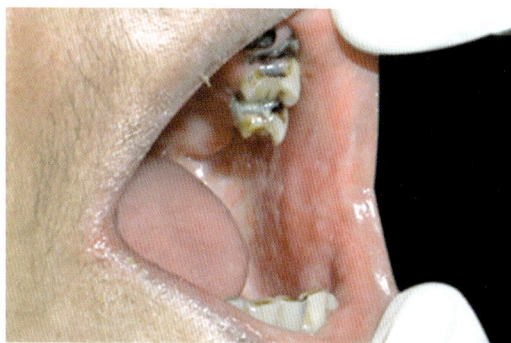

Fig. 2.14: White patchy lesions present on the buccal mucosa: Oral Candidiasis

### *Patient Instructions*

Instructions to resolve this condition, before the construction of new dentures are as follows:
- Clean the old dentures thoroughly with denture cleansers such as hypochlorite or peroxidase
- Avoid night time denture wear to let the tissues breathe
- Trauma due to old dentures needs to be resolved for new dentures to be successful
- Angular chelitis, results in constant dribbling of saliva from the corners of the mouth due to reduced VD with the old dentures. Topical and systemic (if required) medicines need to be administered to combat this fungal infection
- Both the above mentioned problems (trauma due to old dentures and reduced VD) can be temporarily resolved with help of tissue conditioners on the undersurface of the existing dentures till the new dentures are delivered.

## Mucoceles

Poorly adapted dentures with compromised occlusion often result in trauma to the buccal tissues. Constant irritation due to cheek bite during mastication may result in retention cysts and mucoceles. These are chronic mucous retention cysts which need to be excised. Though these cysts are painless they might rupture and recur under the new dentures causing further problems in denture wearers.

## Compromised Tissues

Generalized compromised tissues **(Fig. 2.15)** such as thin atrophic mucosa may not be able to handle even the most perfectly fabricated

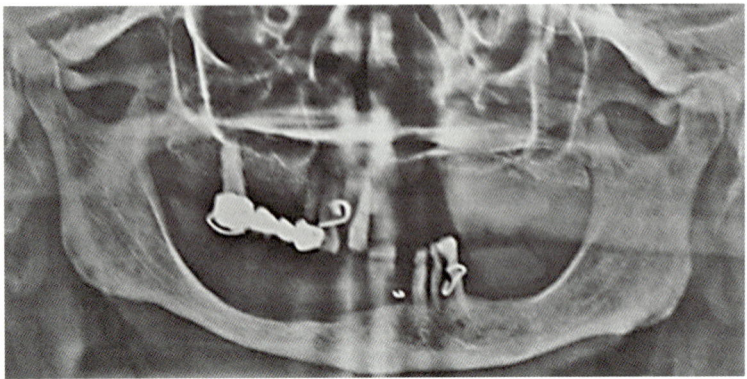

Fig. 2.15: Orthopantomogram: Compromised hard and soft oral tissues in a 75 years old female denture patient

dentures. Such cases can now be handled with less difficulty due to the advent of permanent soft liners **(Fig. 2.16)**. These elastomeric resilient materials are incorporated in complete dentures after the acrylization is complete.

There are two ways to place this soft and flexible material on the intaglio surface of the dentures:
- Chairside procedure
- Laboratory incorporated **(Figs 2.17 and 2.18)**.

The material types and techniques will be discussed in detail in later chapters. Though all the factors for preparing the Oral cavity to accept new complete denture prosthesis are taken into consideration, one of the most important factors is almost always over looked ie: the health and integrity of the hard and soft tissues which will eventually decide the success or failure of a treatment.

Malnourished denture bearing mucosa and underlying bone create a vicious circle causing the mucosa to become thin, friable with extensive bone resorption, resulting in uncomfortable patient and failed prosthesis.

## ■ DENTURE BEARING TISSUES: HEALTH & NUTRITION

A perfectly designed and executed denture may still be termed a failure if the patient is not comfortable with it. Patients suffering from malnourished denture bearing tissues will almost always complain of either tissue irritation or general discomfort. This holds further true due to unfavorable diet in the elderly patients, who are the major recipients of removable prosthesis. Due to reduced physical activity, the need for carbohydrate and fat consumption is minimal in geriatric patients.

## Step 2 Preparation of Oral Cavity

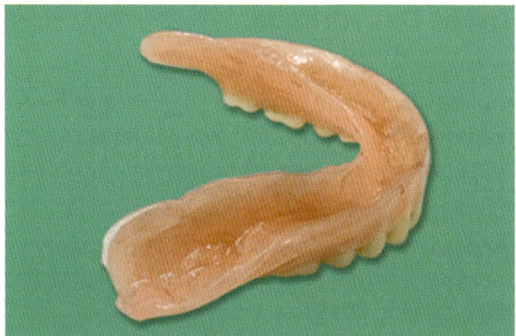

**Fig. 2.16:** Chairside placement of soft liner (Tokuyama tough medium) on a mandibular denture

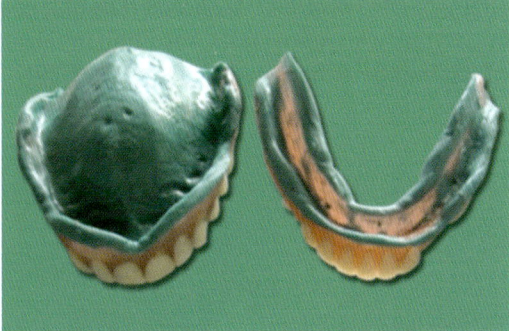

**Fig. 2.17:** Closed mouth impressions made on prefabricated complete dentures to be sent for laboratory relining

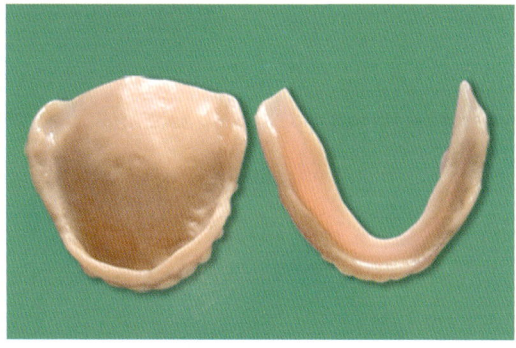

**Fig. 2.18:** Laboratory incorporated relined complete denture prosthesis

It is advisable to consume more proteins and vitamins. Edentulous condition in itself along with loss/reduction of taste sensation results in reduced appetite, inability to chew and enjoy food leading to malnutrition.

As the technician does not come in contact with our patients, it is expected of the clinician to notice and evaluate the nutrition or malnutrition of the tissues. Once the factors are evaluated, the doctor can arrive on a feasible prognosis.

## Tissue Dehydration

*Dryness of mouth:* Xerostomia can compromise any removable prosthesis as the mucous membrane becomes dry and fragile leading to sore spots and loss of denture retention. Artificial saliva and sprays have to be administered for patient comfort.

*Reduction in muscle mass:* Dehydration can result in thinning of muscles, sagging appearance and muscle weakness. Eventually the muscle tone reduces and the prognosis of the prosthesis gets affected **(Fig. 2.19)**.

*Lack of taste sensation:* Accumulation of a coating is very common in patients with xerostomia, resulting in degeneration of taste buds which hampers the sense of taste **(Fig. 2.20)**.

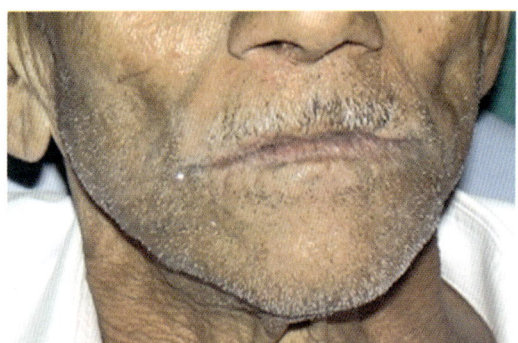

**Fig. 2.19:** Due to reduction in muscle tone and muscle mass: sagging, old appearance of the patient

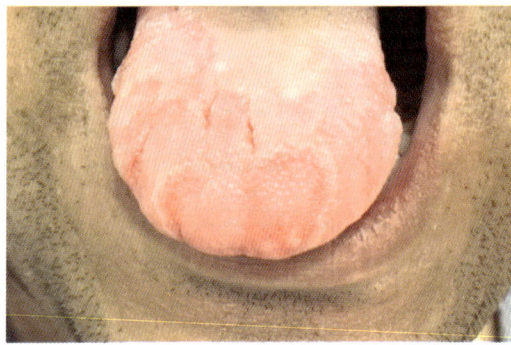

**Fig. 2.20:** Coating and cracks present on the tongue in a patient with xerostomia

## Treatment

Advised increase in fluid intake along with artificial saliva/saliva substitutes in chronic cases. Sugar free candy or lozenges may give temporary relief. Dry mouth patches can also be recommended in severe xerostomia cases as these give relief for 2-4 hours after placement.

## Calcium Deficiency

It may lead to a pathologic condition called Osteoporosis which is characterized by bone loss, mostly of the trabecular bone in weight bearing areas. It is commonly seen in post menopausal women due to hormonal imbalance. Osteoporosis results in increase in bone resorption, weakening of hard supporting tissues and frequent fractures in advanced cases **(Fig. 2.21)**.

## Treatment

Calcium supplements with Vitamin D are included in diet. Low doses of fluoride are indicated as studies prove that it has an important role in remineralization of bone.

## Protein Deficiency

Reduction in protein intake along with increase in carbohydrate ingestion may lead to fatigue, obesity, prevalence of infection and trauma. A marked loss of oral soft tissue elasticity and reduction

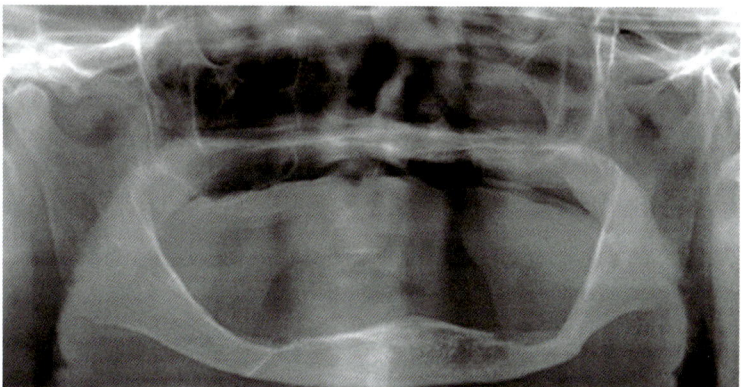

Fig. 2.21: Orthopantomogram: Fracture lines in mandibular jaw due to calcium deficiency and osteoporosis

of masticatory muscle mass and strength results in poor dental prognosis.

***Treatment***

Consumption of food, high in proteins such as pulses, meat and fish.

## Vitamin Depletion

The Vitamins which affect the Oral tissues directly are Vitamin C, Vitamin D and B Complex.

Paucity of these Vitamins can result in following oral conditions:
- Gingival bleeding: Vit C
- Tooth hypermobility: Vit C
- Friable mucosa: Vit C
- Resorbed ridge: Vit D
- Angular chelitis: Vit B12
- Infections such as candidiasis due reduced immunity: Vit C and Vit B-complex.

***Treatment***

Vitamin supplements along with consumption of fresh fruits, juices and vegetables are recommended.

Apart from eating a balanced diet, exercising and taking the required multi vitamin supplements, annual mineral and vitamin deficiency testing can be included along side the regular health check ups.

## Conclusion

- The objectives of complete denture prosthesis are to ascertain functional stability, improved facial appearance, and patient comfort. It is mandatory to evaluate and prepare the oral cavity to ensure that these objectives are satisfactorily met.
- The dentist should consider and recommend pre prosthetic surgical corrections only when all non surgical options have been evaluated.
- If the conditions allow, root support preservation and maintaining stable natural teeth should be a priority.
- Partial/transitional removable dentures aid in patient compliance when future tooth loss is inevitable.

**Step 2** Preparation of Oral Cavity 41

- Due to an increase in life expectancy, patients are likely to retain their natural dentition fairly late in life. The older the patient the more difficult it is for the patient to adjust to a new prosthesis. Therefore good patient doctor communication (explaining the patient role in prosthesis maintenance and limitations of the removable treatment) is necessary during the initial visits.

# Step 3

## Impression Procedures for Dentures

| | | |
|---|---|---|
| 3.1 | Primary Impressions | 43 |
| 3.2 | Final Impressions | 67 |

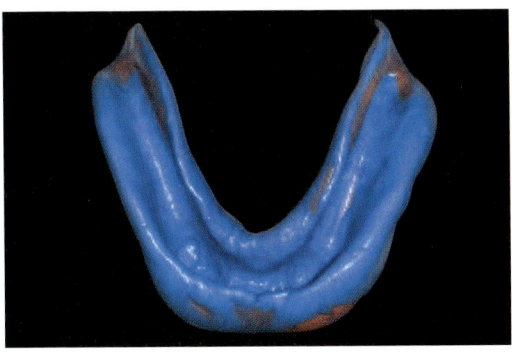

# Step 3.1

## Primary Impressions

*"Perpetual preservation of what remains than the meticulous replacement of what is missing".*
*Muller de Van's dictum*

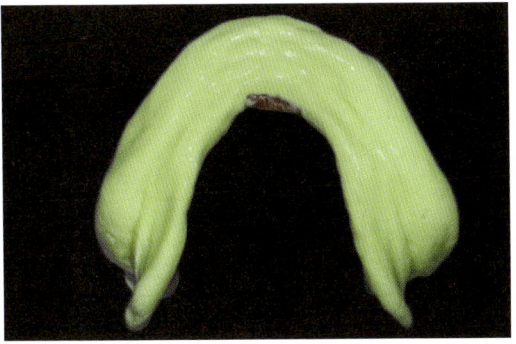

# Step 3.1

# Primary Impressions

## ■ INTRODUCTION

**Aim:** To achieve a satisfactory negative replica of the entire denture bearing area (intaglio surface) **(Fig. 3.1.1)** and the adjacent landmarks for the fabrication of accurately extended custom trays thus ensuring ease of recording a definitive/final impression resulting in perfectly fitting dentures **(Table 3.1.1)**.

**Preservation:** Impression technique and the materials used have a direct effect on the intaglio surface of the denture and eventually on both hard and soft tissues which is reflected in bone resorption and thinning of the mucosa.

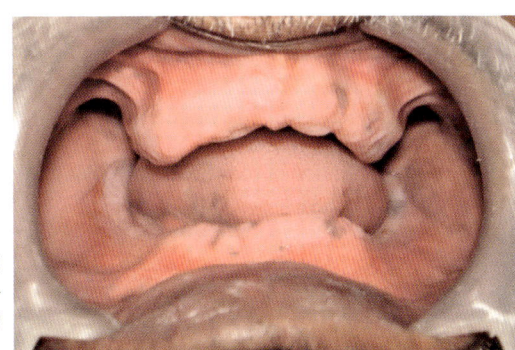

Fig. 3.1.1: Healthy oral tissues: maxillary and mandibular denture bearing areas

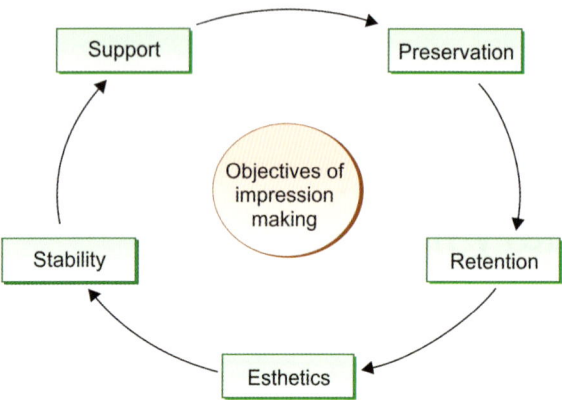

Fig. 3.1.2: Objectives of a perfect impression

**Retention:** Various factors affect retention in a denture. Border retention gets primarily affected by adhesion, cohesion and surface tension helping in peripheral seal. Atmospheric pressure plays a major role in posterior palatal seal.

**Esthetics:** Thickness of the denture is determined by the border thickness while impression making. It varies according to the extent of residual ridge resorption, vestibular sulcus width and depth and the thickness/length of the lips.

**Stability:** It is the resistance to horizontal forces and depends on the type of underlying tissues. A resorbed ridge or flabby tissue will lead to reduced denture stability. A detailed uncompromised recording of the basal seat area with close adaptation increases stability in the prosthesis.

**Support:** Maximum coverage with in the physiological limits to ensure wide distribution of the applied forces is one of the critical objectives of impression making. This is called the "snow shoe

Table 3.1.1: Objectives of impression making

| | |
|---|---|
| P | Preservation of the residual alveolar ridge |
| R | Retention |
| E | Esthetics |
| S | Stability |
| S | Support |

## Step 3.1 Primary Impressions

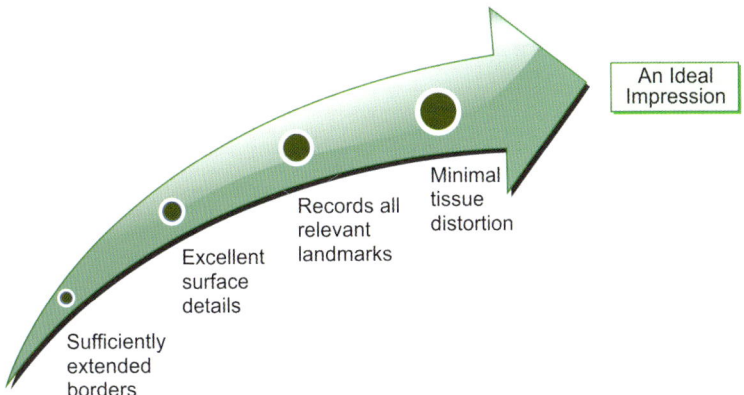

effect", which in turn also aids in preservation, retention and stability of the denture **(Fig. 3.1.2)**.

### ■ REALEFF EFFECT

Complete dentures rest on the alveolar ridge and the oral mucosa which together forms the denture bearing surface or the basal seat area. As the mucosal tissue is movable, compressible and displaceable, Hanau came up with the "realeff effect", i.e. resilience and like effect.

The realeff effect of the mucosa plays a significant role in impression making and the quality of the final dentures. Factors which affect realeff need to be understood such as thin keratinized mucosa, flabby ridge causing displacement of tissues, presence of tissues with fibrous degeneration, denture hyperplasia and others to ensure recording of perfect impressions.

### ■ PRIMARY IMPRESSION: CURRENT CONCEPTS

According to the British Society for the Study of Prosthetic Dentistry (BSSPD), the primary impressions should "accurately record clinically relevant landmarks of the edentulous mouth without excessive tissue distortion" resulting in marginally over extended impressions.

**Step 1:** Complete intraoral examination of the anatomical features of denture bearing area, to be recorded in the primary impression

(**Figs 3.1.3A and B**). Anatomical features of the maxillary and mandibular arch are listed in **Table 3.1.2**.

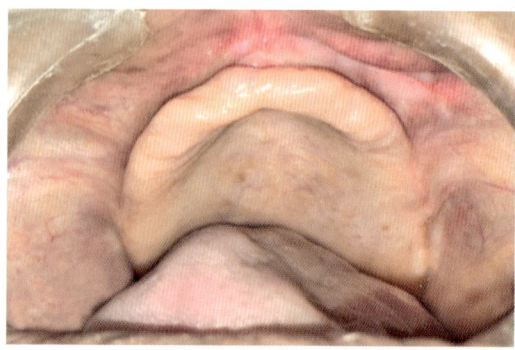

**Fig. 3.1.3A:** Edentulous maxillary arch showing healthy alveolar ridge, free from pathology. Ridge resorption post extraction in maxilla occurs on the buccal aspect of the ridge

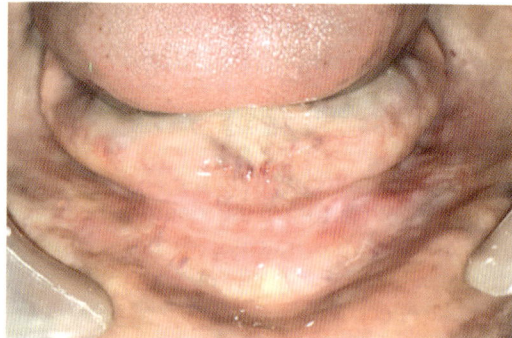

**Fig. 3.1.3B:** Severely resorbed edentulous mandibular ridge. Ridge resorption post extraction occurs mostly on the lingual aspect of the mandibular ridge

**Table 3.1.2:** Anatomical features of maxillary and mandibular arch to be recorded in the primary impression

| Maxillary Arch | Mandibular Arch |
| --- | --- |
| Residual ridge | Residual ridge |
| Maxillary tuberosity and hamular notch | Retromolar pad area |
| Palate: Slopes of palatine shelves with the functional area between hard and soft palate | Lingual frenum, alveolingual sulcus and lingual muscle attachments to the floor of the mouth |
| Vestibular sulci | Vestibular sulci |
| Labial and buccal freni and muscle attachments | Labial and buccal freni |
| Incisive papilla | Mylohyoid ridge |
| Rugae | Retromylohyoid arch |

**Step 2: Choice of materials**—The material to be used for recording primary impressions depends on various factors such as the clinical situation (flabby ridge/residual ridge resorption), doctor's preference, ease of handling and so forth.

The advent of hydrophilic materials revolutionized impression making by increasing the accuracy and enhanced detail reproduction, e.g. alginate and agar-agar. Hydrophobic (moisture / water repellent) materials have various disadvantages, like:
- Poor surface wetting ability
- Low surface detail reproduction
- Inhibit close contact with the basal seat area in presence of saliva.

Other materials which are hydrophobic in nature are compound and silicones. Manufacturers have tried to reduce their hydrophobicity by adding soap like substances called surfactants resulting in more dimensionally stable and water loving impression materials. These materials which have been rendered hydrophilic are called hydroactive. Though hydroactive materials have enhanced affinity for moisture, they do not absorb water like true hydrophilic materials. Thus, these rendered hydrophilic materials are dimensionally extremely stable **(Fig. 3.1.4)**.

The materials most commonly used with predictable results are mentioned in **Table 3.1.3**.

## *Alginate*

Elastic properties make it suitable for recording soft and hard tissue undercuts.

Irreversible hydrocolloid impression material is used in oversized perforated trays. It slumps if not supported by rigid tray material.

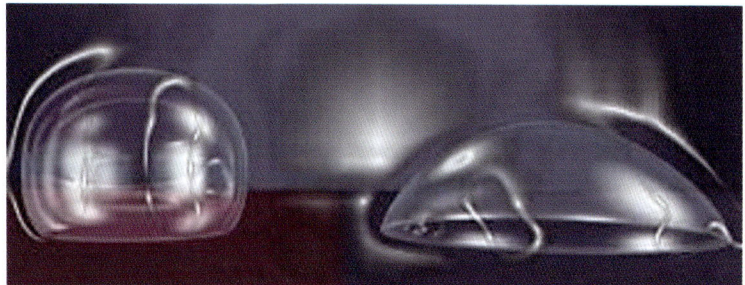

Fig. 3.1.4: Wetting ability of hydrophobic and hydrophilic impression materials

## Procedural Dentistry for Complete Dentures

**Table 3.1.3:** Impression materials of varied consistencies

| Impression Material | Viscosity | Type of Tray Recommended |
|---|---|---|
| Alginate | Light | Perforated, metal/plastic |
| Compound | Viscous | Nonperforated, metal/rigid plastic |
| Heavy body silicon | Medium | Perforated, metal/plastic |
| Putty silicon | Viscous | Perforated/nonperforated, metal/rigid plastic |
| Modified two phase hydrocolloid system | Viscous and light | Perforated, rigid plastic/metal |

Many of the manufacturers have incorporated color changing property in alginate to help the clinicians, i.e. once the mixing time is over the alginate changes color **(Figs 3.1.5A and B)**. This is known as the chromatic phase indicator, which is an indication to load the tray. Mixing time ranges from 30 to 60 seconds.

$$\text{Alginate: Sol} \xrightarrow{\text{Coagulation}} \text{gel}$$

It is mucostatic in nature, i.e. causes minimum tissue displacement. If not poured with in the stipulated time span (20 minutes), it is prone to shrinkage and dimensional instability. Accurate if poured in time, frequently used and cost-effective.

### *Mixing Technique*

- **Conventional hand mixing technique:** A premeasured quantity of water (mL) is placed in a clean flexible rubber bowl. This is followed by the addition of correctly proportioned powder which is sifted in and mixed against the walls of the bowl with a

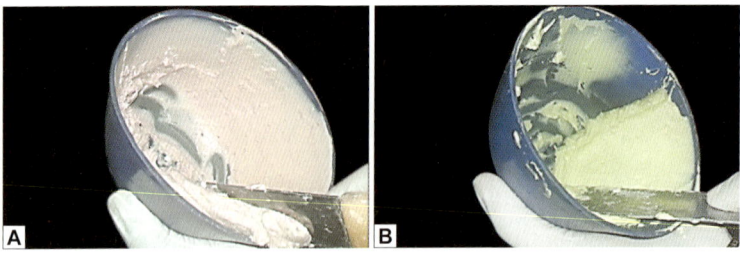

**Figs 3.1.5A and B:** Chromatic alginate is a hydrophilic, irreversible, elastic material which changes colour(from pink to yellow incorporated in this brand) once the mixing time is over. It is an indicator for the clinician to load the tray

wide-blade, curved spatula to reduce air bubble entrapment. A 4:1 (water weight to powder weight) mixing ratio is recommended. The resultant mix should be smooth in consistency but have sufficient body of its own to not drip from the spatula
- **Mechanical machine mixing technique:** A device such as the alginator II (Dux Dental, California) is used to ensure the same quality of alginate mix after every cycle resulting in predictable consistency
- **Two-phase hydrocolloid technique:** The gel of the thinner phase is syringed into the sulci and the viscous phase is loaded onto the tray. The gel is used to record the finer details of the basal seat area where as the viscous phase contributes to the bulk of the impression giving sufficient body to the material, to hold on its own. This technique is developed by Acudent Research and Development Co. Inc., 85 Industrial Way, Buellton, California 93427, USA.

## *Impression Tray Compound*

Reversible thermoplastic material which sets by physical change, commonly used for recording primary impressions. The said material can be reheated and the desired changes made in the impression if needed.

Mucocompressive in nature, i.e. if softened adequately, applies mild to moderate displacement of the tissues during impression making. Low-thermal expansion coefficients resulting in minimal dimensional change make impression compound dimensionally a very stable material.

## *Technique to Mold the Impression Compound*

At the temperature of 54°C, in a heated water bath it loses its rigidity and becomes plastic which can be molded by kneading and then placed in solid metal tray. A thermostatically controlled water bath may be used for the same.

With the advent of newer materials, heavy body and putty elastomers have also been successfully used to record primary impressions.

**Step 3: Selection of impression tray**—The dentist has to choose the correct tray for the patient from an array of preformed trays called stock trays. These are manufactured in a broad range of arch sizes and various forms. Conventionally, the clinician determines the tray size by examining the patient's arch size and placing the tray just distal to the landmark tuberosity for maxillary arch. The tray is rotated inside and lifted anteriorly to visualize the width as well as the length of the tray. The retromolar pad is the landmark for mandibular arch impressions. The different types of stock trays are depicted in **Flowchart 3.1.1**.

A tray compass or a tray selector **(Fig. 3.1.6)** as it is more commonly known is another addition to the clinician's impression making armamentarium. The selector is used to get an approximate idea of the tray size/number appropriate for the patient without placing the trays in the mouth arbitrarily. The tip of the selector is placed bilaterally at the second premolar-molar area of the arch for tray size determination.

**Stock Trays:** Their function is to support the material while impression making and to facilitate impression removal keeping it dimensionally stable, so that a cast can be poured. They are typically either perforated or nonperforated depending on the material to be used. They are further classified as follows:
- Metal-more rigid **(Fig. 3.1.7)**
- Plastic-disposable trays **(Fig. 3.1.8)**
- Thermoplastic—can be altered by dipping in hot water to better suit the anatomy of the maxillary and mandibular arch

*Commonly used materials with preferred stock trays are*
- Alginate: Perforated metal tray with an adhesive is preferred
- Tray compound: Solid metal tray required **(Fig. 3.1.9)**
- Elastomeric silicon: Perforated metal tray preferred.

Flowchart 3.1.1: Types of stock trays

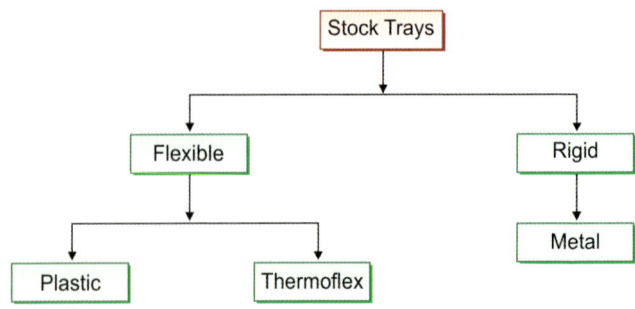

## Step 3.1 Primary Impressions

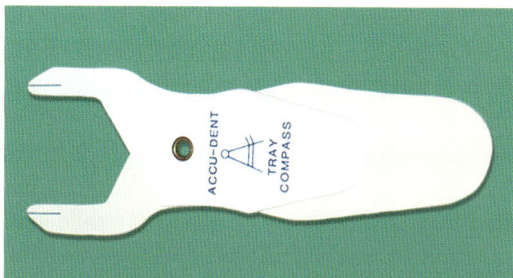

Fig. 3.1.6: Tray selector/Tray compass: Helps to get an approximate idea of the stock tray size to be used

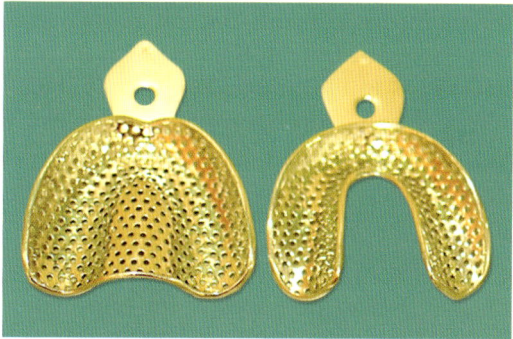

Fig. 3.1.7: Perforated, rigid, metal stock trays

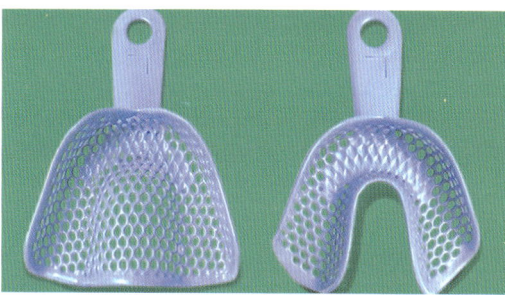

Fig. 3.1.8: Plastic disposable stock trays

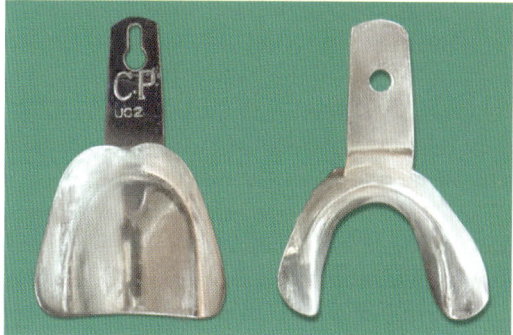

Fig. 3.1.9: Solid, non perforated, rigid, metal stock trays

A perforated tray is used with a hydrocolloid like alginate. The vents allow the material to lock the impression in place once it is set by providing mechanical retention. As alginate is less dimensionally stable compared to tray compound or even silicon like heavy body and putty, these perforations along with retention provide stability.

Once the stock tray and the material have been selected, the material is loaded on to the tray while the clinician adjusts his position to one side and behind the patient for maxillary and in front of the patient for the mandibular.

**Maxillary impression:** The tray is rotated in and held anteriorly first to record the labial sulcus and incisive papilla, then placed backwards to fill the buccal vestibule. Finally, the palatal area is recorded as the tray is pressed into position.

**Mandibular impression:** The tray is inserted and placed over the alveolar ridge. Once in position the loaded tray is lowered towards the buccal vestibule posteriorly and then pressed forward to record the anterior portion of the ridge and labial vestibule.

**Step 4: Patient preparation for impressioning**—Each and every patient is unique. They have their fears and problems which cannot be always clubbed into a category. Therefore, a thorough oral examination and check of the oral cavity for anatomical variations such as deep palate, maxillary/mandibular tori, resorbed or flabby residual ridge, etc. is done. It is imperative at this stage to find out more about the patient's individual difficulties such as gag response, saliva thickness, dryness of the mouth and even the psychological impact of being edentulous has on the patient.

It is also recommended to discuss the procedure with the patient to ensure compliance, ease and enhance patient comfort.

For the lower impression, patient is seated in an upright position with the mandible parallel to the floor. Doctor stands in front of the patient, i.e. facing the patient **(Fig. 3.1.10)** before inserting the tray in a way, that one side of the tray enters the mouth before the other side follows. This way the surrounding tissues such as the lips and cheeks do not get over stretched.

For recording the upper impression, patient's head is lifted / tilted to an angle where the maxillary arch gets parallel to the floor. Doctor stands just behind and sideways at 11 o'clock position as the tray is rotated in the mouth for ease of placement **(Fig. 3.1.11)**.

## Step 3.1 Primary Impressions

**Step 5: Preparing the oral cavity just before impression making—** Once the patient is seated correctly with the occiput/head resting on the head rest the impression material is prepared according to the manufacturer's instructions. The patient is asked to rinse the mouth with cold water to wash away most of the saliva from the oral cavity. For those patients with abundant thick ropey saliva, it is preferable to place an astringent mouth wash in the rinsing water to reduce viscosity of saliva. Cold water also reduces the gag reflex in some patients which usually gets triggered during maxillary impression making.

**Step 6: Impressions**

**Maxillary arch:** After selecting a correct size tray, utility wax or any other variant such as compound or greenstick may be used for tray extensions along the borders and posterior palatal seal area if required. For a high palate, it may also be added on the center of the tray to help in recording the impression without voids. Mix the material adequately as discussed and fill the tray beginning

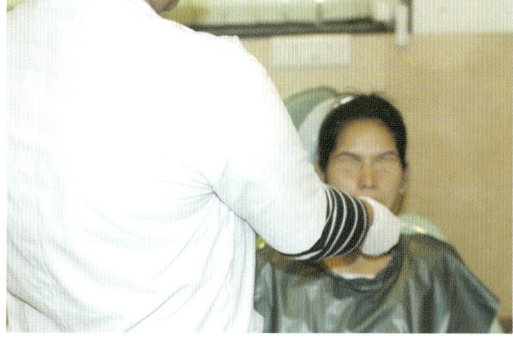

Fig. 3.1.10: For the mandibular impression: Patient is seated upright with the mandible parallel to the floor. Doctor stands in front facing the patient

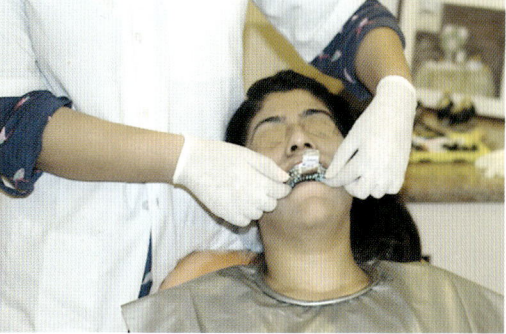

Fig. 3.1.11: For the maxillary impression, patient's head is lifted to an angle making the maxillary arch parallel to the floor. Doctor stands just behind and sideways at 11 o'clock position

from one side to the other to prevent air entrapment. The tray once rotated in, is first lowered anteriorly to record the incisive papilla, anterior palate with the vestibule, then pressed posteriorly. Patient is asked to tilt the head down so the maxilla gets parallel to the floor and to take short breaths through the nose. This will relax the palatal muscles which help in recording the posterior palatal seal area. The freni are relieved **(Fig. 3.1.12)** as the labial and buccal sulcus is molded by manipulating the lip and cheek area for a great impression.

**Mandibular arch:** The selected tray is refined at the alveololingual and the posterior border with the help of extension materials. As the tray is loaded, patient is asked to rinse the mouth. Ideally, the tray is lowered posteriorly to record the retromolar pad area and then it is pressed anteriorly to complete the seating of the impression. Once the tray is firmly seated, the patient is asked to raise the tongue and keep it anteriorly to record the alveololingual sulcus while the clinician molds the labial and buccal area.

For more rigid materials like impression compound **(Figs 3.1.13A and B)** all the movements are exaggerated including recording the freni. In mandibular impression the patient moves the tongue sideways as well. The acceptable maxillary and mandibular primary impressions recorded with alginate are shown in **Figures 3.1.14A and B)**.

**Step 7:** **Checking the quality of the impression**—Many clinicians feel that an imperfect primary impression in denture fabrication is acceptable as the faults will get rectified in the secondary impression. This is wrong. Failure to record a good primary impression will lead

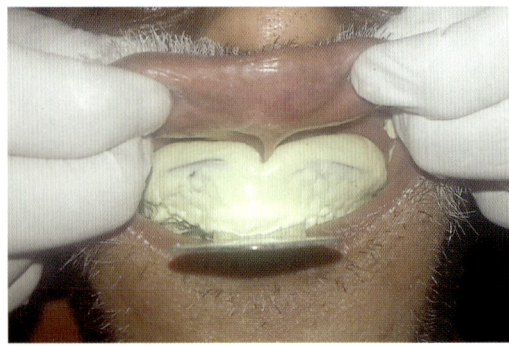

Fig. 3.1.12: Labial frenum is relieved in the maxillary primary impression

## Step 3.1 Primary Impressions

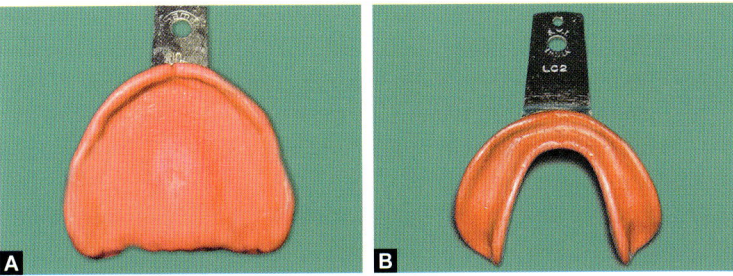

**Figs 3.1.13A and B:** Acceptable maxillary and mandibular impressions recorded with Impression compound

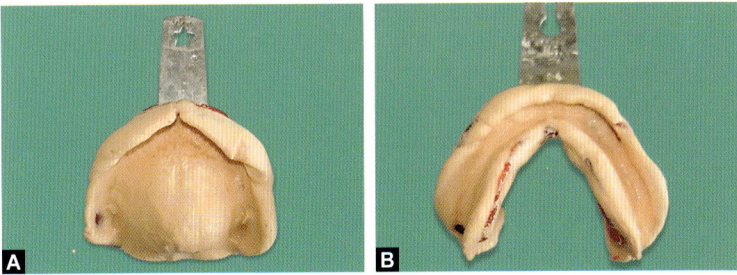

**Figs 3.1.14A and B:** Acceptable maxillary and mandibular primary impressions recorded with alginate

to an unacceptable secondary impression, which in turn will result in poor dentures and unhappy patients.

## Dysfunctional Impressions

What is not acceptable?
- Tray exposure: This occurs due to the following causes:
  - Improper seating of tray
  - Excessive finger pressure on the tray
  - Over extended tray.
- Distorted impression:
  - Early retrieval of the loaded tray
  - Inadequate tray size
  - Impression tray incorrectly centered
  - Forward thrust by the tongue can impact the stability of the tray while impression is setting in the oral cavity.
- Rough, uneven and glossy/dull surface with voids (**Fig. 3.1.15**)

- Incorrect handling of the material by the clinician/assistant/laboratory personal
- Inability to adhere to the manufacturer's instruction
- Failure to manipulate rigid materials while seating the tray causing inadequate molding of the tissues, e.g. impression compound.

• Insufficient anatomical details such as cleft or a fissure in mid palatine region or flat alveololingual sulcus:
- Insufficient material placed in the stock tray
- Under extended tray resulting in slumping of the materials like alginate
- Insufficient heating/softening of the rigid materials like compound leads to inadequate recording of denture bearing area
- Inadequate seating pressure on the tray
- Tongue getting trapped under the flanges while seating the mandibular impression.

**Step 8: Disinfection**—As a protocol it is mandatory that each and every impression must be disinfected before, either pouring the impression at the clinic or sending it to the laboratory to prevent cross infection. If disinfection of the impression is not done the correct way, the gypsum cast will become contaminated and is capable of acting as a vector for propagation of infection/germ transmission to the dental assistants, technicians, transporting persons and all those who handle the set impression/cast. According to studies set impressions are a source of infection due to presence of microorganisms such as bacteria, virus and fungi. Some of these may be pathogenic in nature such as mycobacterium tuberculi.

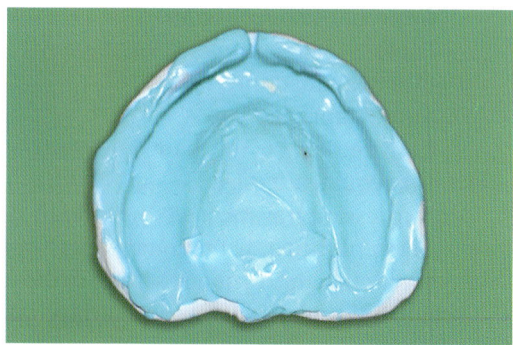

Fig. 3.1.15: Dysfunctional impression: Though elastomeric impression material has been used, the impression is distorted and has discrepancies such as air bubbles and material drag

## Step 3.1 Primary Impressions

**According to British Dental Association's infection control guide:** "The only safe approach to routine treatment is to assume that every patient may be a carrier of an infectious disease". Thus, the need of disinfecting all impressions.

A huge array of methods and materials have been used in the past and quoted in literature for the purpose of disinfection/sterilization of impressions. The ones discussed here, are those which are most commonly used by clinicians and have withstood the test of time emerging as definite winners.

The most common modes are as follows:
- Disinfectant sprays
- Solutions
- Ethylene oxide gas sterilization.

### Disinfectants Used

- 0.5% sodium hypochlorite
- 2% glutaraldehyde.
- Isopropyl alcohol spray
- Peracetic acid
- Iodophores.

### Disinfection Procedures Using Solutions/Sprays

- Cleaning of impression by rinsing to get rid of blood, saliva and debri (bioburden)
- The set impression is then disinfected by either immersing the impression in the aforementioned disinfectant for approximately 10 minutes
- Rinsing is carried out after disinfecting the impression under running water, to remove the traces of the chemical from the impression. Failure to do so can result in substandard casts and eventually a failed prosthesis.

All the elastomers, impression tray compound are easily disinfected using the immersion technique without the fear of dimensional instability. However hydrocolloids react differently.

Alginates if immersed, then should be removed within a minute and placed in a sealed plastic bag for the remaining time period. Once the recommended 10 minutes are over, it is cleaned thoroughly.

- Spraying the impression with a disinfectant is a popular option. After spraying, the impression should be kept in a sealed bag for 10 minutes
- The impression may be wrapped in a disinfectant soaked cloth prior to placing the impression in a sealed container.

Ideally, during each and every step of denture construction the clinician should adhere to strict disinfection protocol.

**Step 9: Storage**—Dimensionally stable materials like elastomers and compound do not pose any difficulty in storage. On the other hand alginate impressions need to be poured immediately. It is important to understand the storage protocol for irreversible hydrocolloids, if they need to be stored for either pouring at a later time or have to be transferred to the laboratory for the same. The storage should be at 100% relative humidity in a plastic ziplock bag or wrapped under damp gauze till poured.

**Step 10: Pouring the cast**—Once the clinician is satisfied with the quality of the impression and the disinfection procedure has been followed, the impression is ready for pouring.

**Do's:** To protect the borders of the impression and the finer details, it is beaded and then boxed with the beading and boxing wax **(Fig. 3.1.16)** respectively. The stone can be either hand mixed or vacuum mixed. The latter is used to avoid air entrapment in the mix which is ultimately poured using vibrating machine for cast fabrication. The mixing time is around 30–40 seconds depending on the speed of the automatic mixer.

**Don't's:** Commonly the primary impression is turned upside down during pouring onto the base of stone/plaster. This mistake results

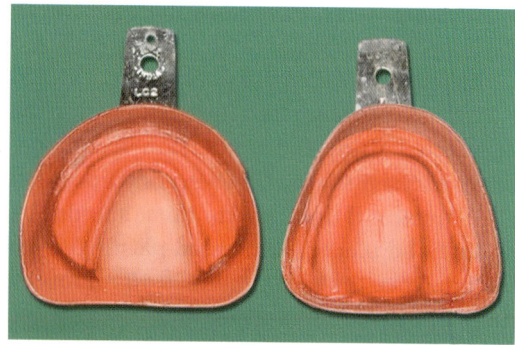

Fig. 3.1.16: Beaded and boxed primary impressions recorded with impression compound. It is done to protect the borders and the finer details of the impression

in soft outer layer of the cast due to settling of thin watery stone mix at the surface forming faulty, unusable casts.

Before pouring, the impression should be sprinkled with dental stone/plaster to bind with remaining free alginic acid. This powder is then washed away with water and then finally poured. The poured cast should be separated from the impression as soon as the stone is adequately set to prevent moth-eaten appearance with some materials **(Fig. 3.1.17)**.

## TIPS "N" TRICKS TO AVOID COMMON MISTAKES WHILE MAKING PRELIMINARY IMPRESSIONS

- When mixing alginate for a primary impression, it is preferable to dispense less water than usual quantity as that will result in a more viscous putty like consistency of the mixture. In most of the cases this results in reduced gag reflex and better handling of the material
- A thicker mix of alginate will also give better impressions as a loose mix gets further thinned out at the borders in the vestibular area due to heavy muscle trimming
- While making impressions with compound one must consider the thermoplastic nature of the material. The slightly warmer oral cavity causes the surface layer of the compound impression to remain softer in comparison to the body of the impression. The cooling starts from the base that is in contact with the tray. Therefore, it should be left in the mouth a little longer than the setting time dictates
- The loaded compound impression tray should not be submerged completely in warm water during impression correction or

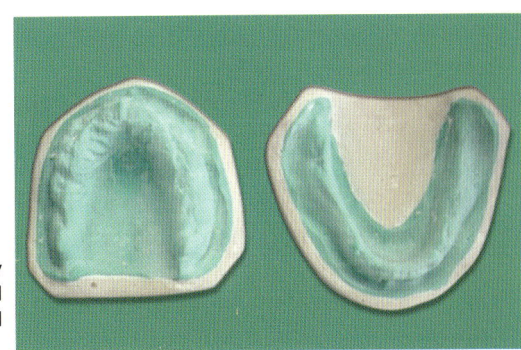

**Fig. 3.1.17:** Primary casts poured in dental stone with a dental plaster base

manipulation. The compound attached to the tray needs to maintain shape
- If alginate is to be used with nonperforated stock trays then a hydrocolloid adhesive is mandatory to prevent impression from detaching from the tray
- In patients with unmanageable thick, excessive saliva a simple rinsing protocol is to be followed. First make the patient rinse with warm water which opens the salivary gland ducts and allows the saliva to flow out. Then rinsing with cold water mixed with astringent as it will constrict the duct openings and thin down the present saliva in the oral cavity making the impressioning simpler
- For recording a deep palatal vault: It is useful to modify the tray by placing utility wax on the center of the tray helping the impression material to record the palate. Placing some impression material directly on the palate at the time of impression making also results in good impressions without voids. Same can be done if deep sulci are present
- Always practice the insertion of the stock tray without loading the tray to check tray dimensions as well as for ensuring patient compliance
- Remember, working and setting time are higher during increase in humidity and temperature of the surroundings
- Depending on the anatomy of the soft tissues of the denture bearing area, the material can be chosen, e.g. compound used only if the tissue is firm with little mobility. If the tissue is flabby or movable then alginate is preferred as it records the impression with minimal displacement
- In patients with high gag reflex, where we do not want the trouble of the water bath, silicon (putty consistency) can also be used with ease
- Never use a moist/wet spatula to take alginate powder out of the box/packet. This will lead to a chain reaction where the powder in those areas starts to set leading to grainy mix and inaccurate impressions. It will also affect the working and the setting time
- To prevent distortion/loosening of the impression in the areas where there is less support from the tray such as the posterior or distobuccal areas, the impression should always be stored with the open area facing downward

## Step 3.1 Primary Impressions

- A poured alginate impression should never be left overnight without separating the cast from the impression. The contraction of the material due to loss of water can lead to difficulty in impression separation and breakage of thinner parts of the cast resulting in cast inaccuracy.

## Conclusion

- A primary impression must record the complete denture bearing area with accuracy. A low quality preliminary impression if accepted will lead to a substandard final impression compromising denture retention and stability.
- Clinicians use various materials to record primary impressions. The impression reproducing sulcus depth, sulcus width along the periphery and important anatomical landmarks is acceptable, irrelevant to the type of material used to record the same.

# Step 3.2

## Final Impressions

*"Complete denture educational programs agree on many aspects of final impression making, however, there is variability in their teachings regarding the impression philosophy and the materials used."*

                                                                Petropoulosetal

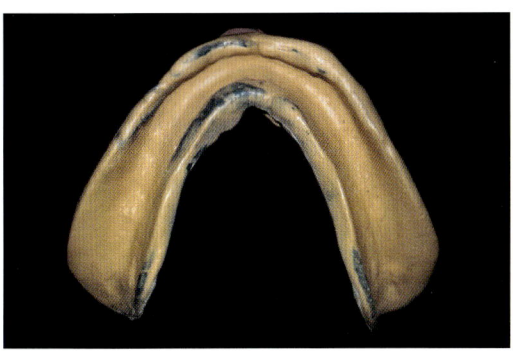

# Step 3.2

# Final Impressions

## ■ INTRODUCTION

A satisfactory final impression needs to be resistant to displacement of the dentures away from the denture bearing area, towards the tissues or against the lateral forces which displace the dentures in a side to side or antero posterior direction. A good retentive denture is fabricated when these five objectives are fulfilled:

1. **Retention:** Resist displacement of the dentures away from the basal seat area. Ex: Sticky food.
2. **Stability:** Resist displacement of the dentures laterally or anteroposteriorly. Ex: Flabby tissues, Residual ridge resorption.
3. **Support:** Resist displacement of the dentures towards the denture bearing tissues. Ex: Maximum tissue coverage within the physiologic limits.
4. **Preservation:** Ensure relief areas are maintained and bone loss is kept at a minimum during function. Ex: incisive palillae, thin resorbed ridge.
5. **Comfort and Esthetics:** Patient acceptance of the new denures is directly proportional to the comfort level which goes hand in hand with how esthetically pleasing the denture is. Ex: sore spot elimination, bulky dentures.

Compromising even one objective can result in unretentive dentures. For example, if there is sufficient suction/retention achieved in a denture but the occlusion is compromised, the denture may lose retention due to instability.

The success of a retentive complete denture prosthesis depends on the factors which influence the dimension and shape of the borders of the final impression **(Fig. 3.2.1)**. The final structure of the peripheral roll is mainly dependent upon the activity of muscle attachments in the area. Muscles of Modiolus affect the border molding and the final impression. It is a fibromuscular mass, bluntly cone shaped and a diameter of 4 × 10 × 20 mm with kidney shaped modiolar base **(Fig. 3.2.2)**.

## Custom Tray Fabrication

A custom tray is fabricated after a satisfactory primary impression has been recorded. A spacing of 0.5-1 mm (space for the final impression material) is achieved in the acrylic custom tray with the help of a spacer wax **(Figs 3.2.3A and B)**. This tray is seated in the oral cavity and extensions are checked. The tray can be fabricated by either light cure, or self cure techniques. Self cure technique is more commonly used whereas light cure is the easiest.

### *Maxillary Custom Tray Border Extension Checklist*

- After placing the tray in the oral cavity, there should be 2-4 mm clearance between the tray and the vestibular sulcus. Two mm space for green stick material where as 3-4 mm clearance if heavy body or soft putty silicon is used for border molding **Figures 3.2.4 and 3.2.5)**
- Similar clearance is checked in all the frenal attachments **(Fig. 3.2.6)**. Overextended areas to be trimmed and if grossly under extended then the tray is discarded and another fabricated
- Posterior extension correlated with the posterior vibrating line by asking the patient to say "aah". Once the anterior and posterior vibrating lines are delineated in the oral cavity, the posterior limit of the custom tray is marked according to the posterior vibrating line. This will be the limit of the posterior extension in the final denture **(Fig. 3.2.7)**.

### *Mandibular Custom Tray Border Extension Checklist*

- The tray is placed and checked to ensure that there is enough clearance (2-4 mm) all around the tray borders and sulcus including the areas of frenum attachment
- In the alveolo-lingual sulcus, the tray must be 1-2 mm below the mylohyoid ridge to eliminate impingement during lateral movement in the final denture base
- Posteriorly, the tray should cover the retro-mylohyoid area as this will help in creating a border seal for denture retention

## Step 3.2  Final Impressions

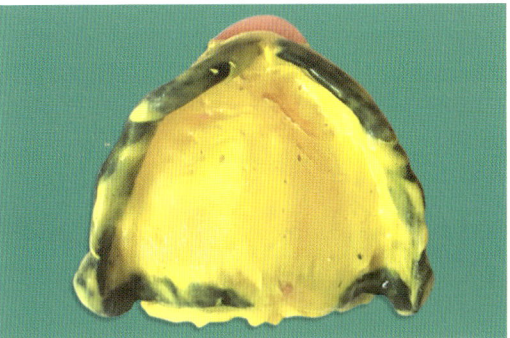

Fig. 3.2.1: Final impression utilizing green stick compound for border molding and light body addition silicon (Honigum, DMG) for the wash impression. Notice the peripheral roll needed for a successful impression

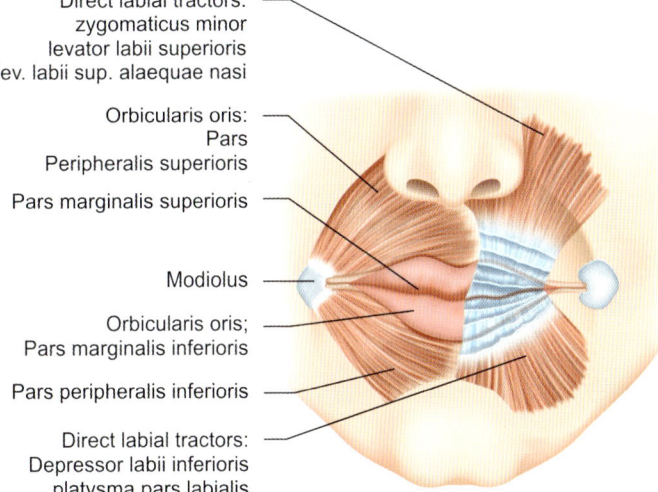

Fig. 3.2.2: Muscles affecting the impression registration: Muscles of modiolus

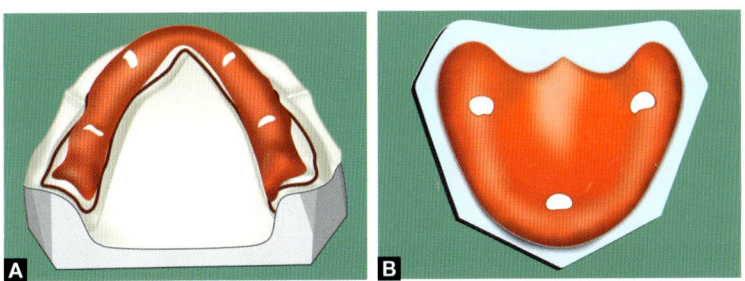

Figs 3.2.3A and B: Spacer wax placement on mandibular and maxillary cast

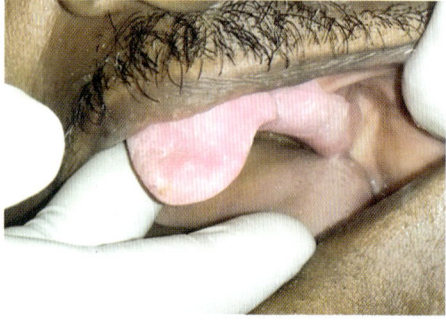

Fig. 3.2.4: 2-4mm clearance checked between the custom tray and the vestibular area: Left side

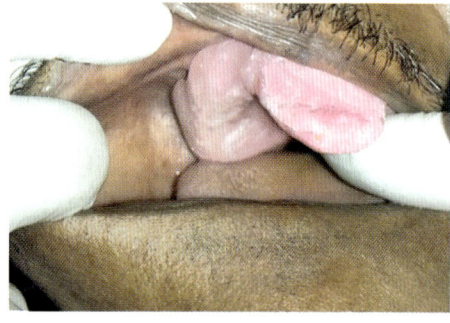

Fig. 3.2.5: 2-4mm clearance checked between the custom tray and the vestibular area: Right side

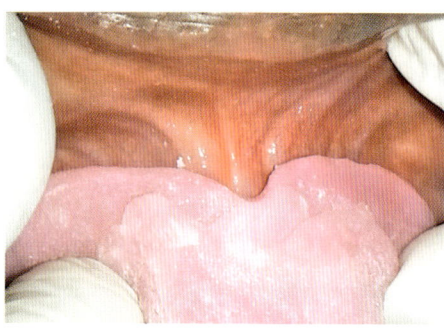

Fig. 3.2.6: Clearance for the labial frenum checked in relation the custom tray

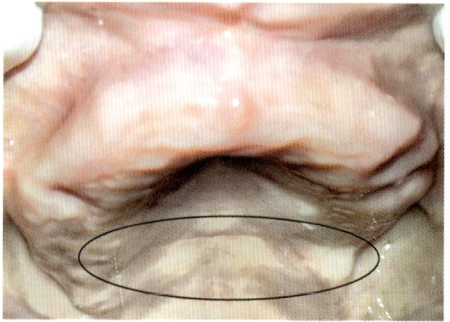

Fig. 3.2.7: Posterior denture extension visible as a line in existing or old denture wearers

**Step 3.2** Final Impressions

### Setting Process of Custom Tray Materials

| | |
|---|---|
| Cold cure set: Original old school materials which set by chemical reaction and produce heat while setting: Exothermic reaction. Chances of warpage are high **(Fig. 3.2.8)**. | 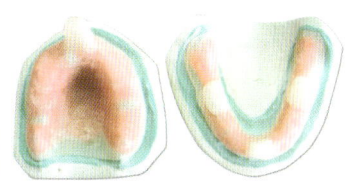<br>**Fig. 3.2.8:** Cold cure acrylic custom trays |
| Light cure set: Once the soft uncured tray material is placed on the cast and adjusted to the desired shape and dimension, the material is placed in a UV chamber for 2-3 minutes where it hardens. Easy handling and dimensional stability is exceptional **(Figs 3.2.9A and B)**. | 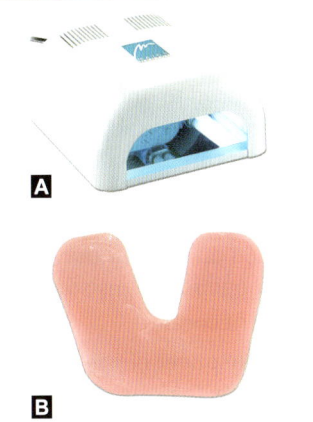<br>**Figs 3.2.9A and B:** (A) Light unit for curing the light cure custom trays. (B) Light cure tray material |
| Cold cure set- Polymorph: Newer thermoplastic material. The beads are manipulated into a dough which is placed on to the cast and shaped into a custom tray. After the excess is cut the material is placed under cold water for final set. Easy to use with good adaptation and stability **(Figs 3.2.10A and B)**. | 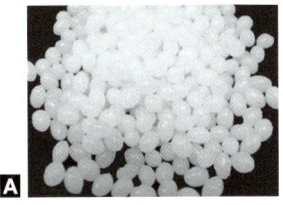<br>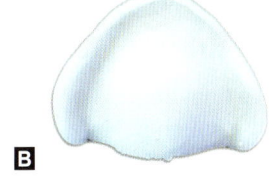<br>**Figs 3.2.10A and B:** (A) Polymorph beads. (B) Custom tray with cold cure polymorph beads |

## Materials Used for Border Molding and Final Impression

Green stick tracing compound is one of the most commonly used materials for recording border extensions **(Fig. 3.2.11)**. But, with advent of newer materials, silicon in various consistencies such as heavy body, functional silicon impression material **(Figs 3.2.12A and B)** and soft putty, these have become the materials of choice in many clinical practices. There are various advantages of using silicon over green stick compound:
- Time advantage: The total time in border molding comes down to 3-5 mts depending on the setting time of the material
- Single shot border molding: The number of insertions of the tray is reduced to one
- Superior accuracy: Reduction in error propagation as all the borders are recorded simultaneously
- Water bath elimination
- Ease of manipulation/handling: Silicon is kneadable and can be placed on the tray borders with ease and no slumping
- Homogenous consistency
- Patient comfort.

Zinc oxide eugenol impression paste **(Figs 3.2.13A and B)** though still used by various clinicians due to its properties of dimensional stability and replicating surface details, has taken a back seat as more and more dentists are using light body silicon impression material. Reasons for the decline of Zinc oxide eugenol paste as an impression material:
- Burning sensation causes discomfort to the patient
- Locks in deep undercut areas and is extremely difficult to disengage resulting in breakage/fracture of the recorded final impression in that area
- Eugenol allergy in some patients
- Messy to work with as it adheres to instruments and face making it difficult to clean.

## Final Impression Technique

Ideally, a final impression technique should follow selective pressure theory by Boucher. Here, certain areas such as incisive papilla in the maxilla and sharp resorbed ridge in the mandible, which need to be relieved, have reduced pressure due to vents created in those areas in the custom tray. The borders of the tray record the shape of the sulcus in function accurately to ensure a satisfactory peripheral seal.

## Step 3.2 Final Impressions

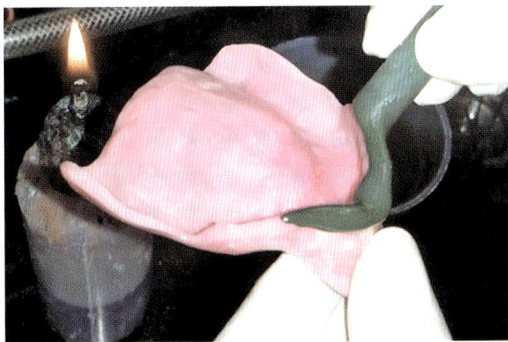

Fig. 3.2.11: Green stick tracing compound being applied for sectional border molding

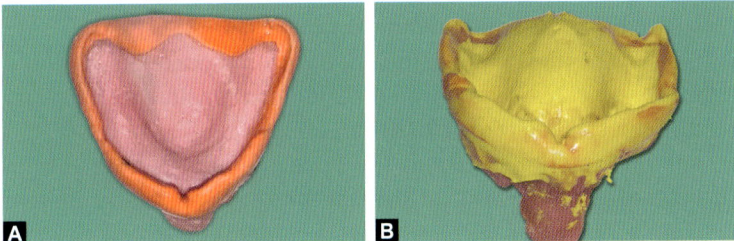

Figs 3.2.12A and B: (A) Single shot border molding with functional silicon impression material. (B) Final impression with light body silicon impression material

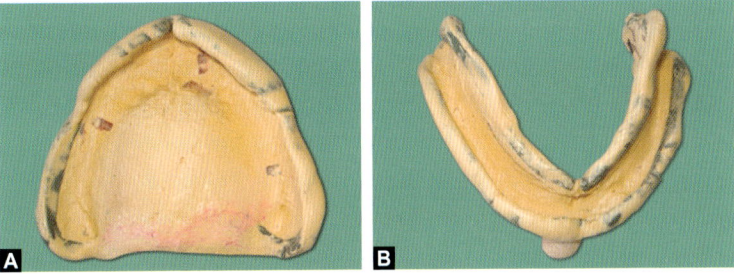

Figs 3.13A and B: Final impression recorded with Zinc oxide eugenol paste. It is still the most commonly used final impression material in the country

Once the tray extensions are verified, the custom tray is ready for border molding. If green stick tracing compound is used then there are various insertions whereas with silicon the number of insertions is as low as one. Whichever material is used, the movements and the technique remains the same. The only difference is, that for silicons an adhesive has to be applied before placing the material on the tray as they do not have inherent adhesive properties.

## Maxillary Tray Border Molding

- Material is added to the tray border either in part, in a sequential manner for green stick or at one go for silicon
- For maxillary posterior/buccal area the flange is molded by extending the cheek outward, downward and inward which follows the muscle movements **(Fig. 3.2.14)**
- Patient is asked to pucker and smile
- In the buccal freni area the cheek is again extended outward, downward, inward and also moved backward and forward to replicate the frenii movement **(Figs 3.2.15, 3.2.16 and 3.2.17)**
- Patient is asked to open the mouth wide and then close to create space for the pterygomandibular raphae **(Fig. 3.2.18)**
- Side to side movement of the jaw to accommodate the coronoid notch which is seen as a small indentation in the maxillary distobuccal area **(Fig. 3.2.19)**
- For the anterior area and the labial frenum, elevate the lip upward and downward. Massage the lip with lateral motion **(Figs 3.2.20 and 3.2.21)**
- Patient is asked to say aah and the posterior vibrating line observed. This is where the final impression and eventually the denture should end
- Aah, swallowing or Valsalva's maneuver (Close the patients nose and ask him to push air through the nose causing the posterior palatal area to lift) with the head bowed down to record the Posterior palatal seal area **(Fig. 3.2.22)**.

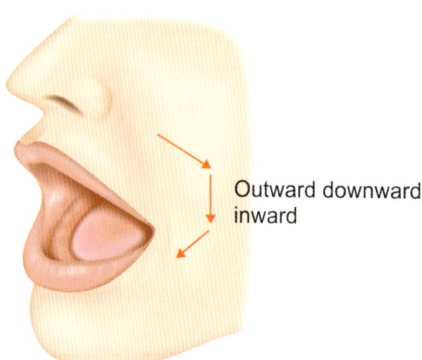

**Fig. 3.2.14:** The flange is molded by extending the cheek outward, downward and inward for maxillary arch buccal area

## Step 3.2 Final Impressions

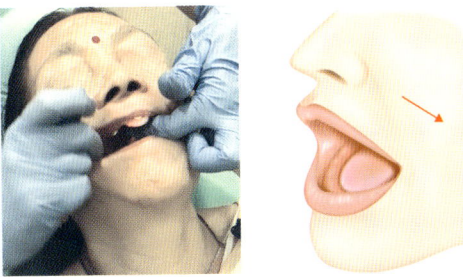

Fig. 3.2.15: Cheek extended outward

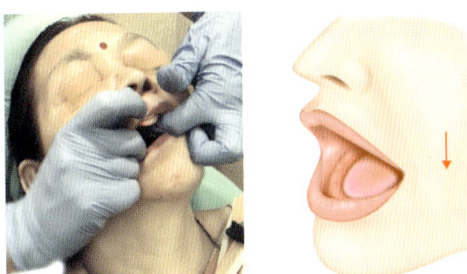

Fig. 3.2.16: Cheek extended downward

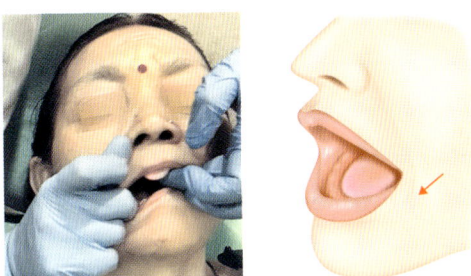

Fig. 3.2.17: Cheek extended inward

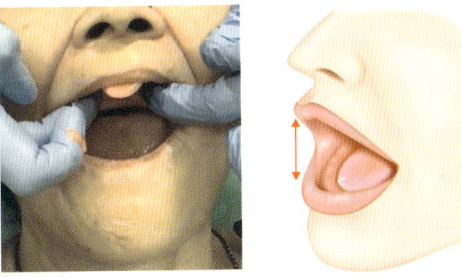

Fig. 3.2.18: Patient is asked to open the mouth wide

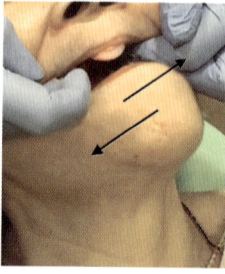 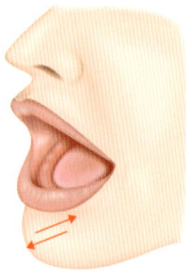

Fig. 3.2.19: Side to side movement of the lower jaw

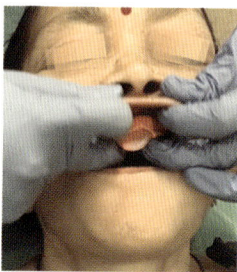 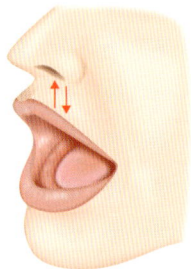

Fig. 3.2.20: For the anterior area and the labial frenum, elevate the lip upward and downward

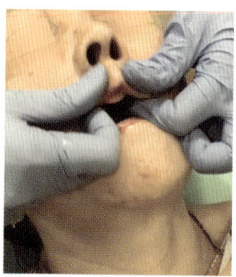 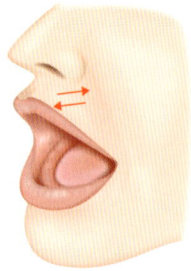

Fig. 3.2.21: Massage the lip with lateral motion

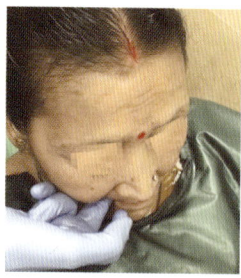 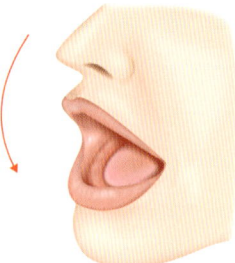

Fig. 3.2.22: The head bowed down to record the posterior palatal seal area

## Mandibular Tray Border Molding

- For mandibular buccal area the flange is molded outward, upward and inward to replicate muscle movements whereas backward and forward movements are done to record the frenii **(Fig. 3.2.23)**
- Patient is asked to purse the lips and smile to simulate the muscular movement
- Muscle activity in anterior flange with frenum is replicated by gently lifting the lower lip outward, upward and inward
- Patient is told to close/clench the mouth while the clinician puts pressure in the opposite direction (tries to open). This activates the masseter muscle which pushes against the buccinator resulting in the formation of massetric notch in the mandibular disto buccal area **(Fig. 3.2.24)**
- If it is ignored, the pressure can result in loss of denture retention

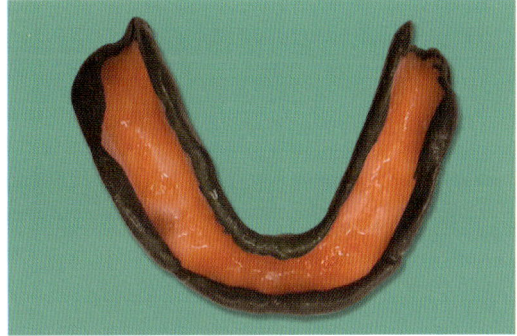

Fig. 3.2.23: Mandibular tray border molding utilizing sectional technique with green stick tracing compound

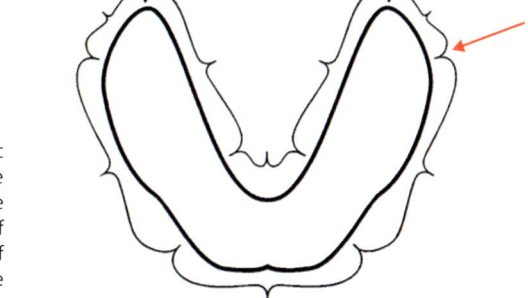

Fig. 3.2.24: Massetric notch is recorded in the disto buccal area of the mandibular impression. If ignored can cause loss of denture retention while chewing

- Anterior lingual flange: patient is asked to protrude the tongue out which determines the length of the lingual flange and to push against the anterior palate for recording the flange thickness.
- Side to side/lateral tongue movement will record the complete alveolo-lingual sulcus **(Fig. 3.2.25)**.

As a retentive border molded tray is achieved, it is ready for final impression. The spacer wax is removed and 1 mm diameter vents are created. Vents are placed strategically in areas to reduce/remove pressure points and create relief.

The areas where vents are created are as follows:
- Maxillary tray **(Fig. 3.2.26)**:
    - Incisive papilla
    - Mid palatine raphe
    - Center of palatine shelves.
- Mandibular tray:
    - On the height of the alveolar ridge **(Fig. 3.2.27)**.

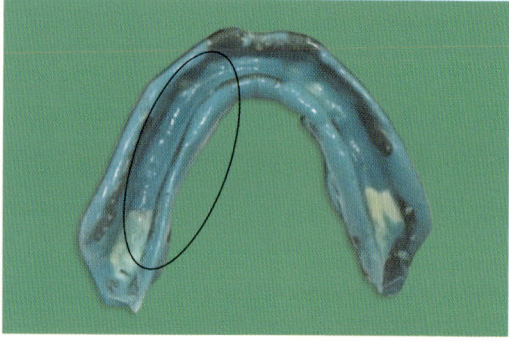

Fig. 3.2.25: Mandibular impression recording the complete alveolingual sulcus. It is the space recorded between the mandibular alveolar ridge and the lateral aspect of the tongue

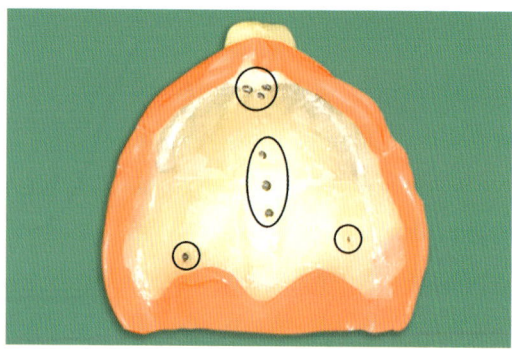

Fig. 3.2.26: Placement of vents in the maxillary tray

## Step 3.2 Final Impressions

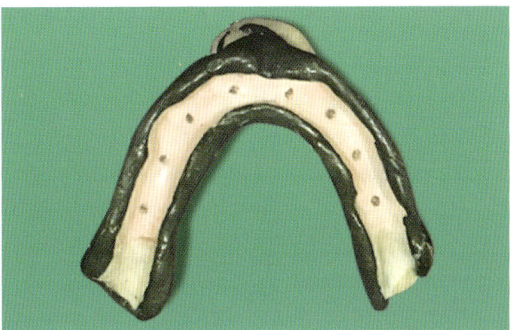

Fig. 3.2.27: Placement of vents in the mandibular tray

### *Purpose of the Vents*

- Permit proper seating of the tray
- Helps in relief of certain areas
- Prevents air entrapment and bubble formation in the final impression **(Fig. 3.2.28)**
- Better flow of the material.

The final impression material is spread all over the border molded tray. The clinician must ensure that the borders are also covered with the low viscosity impression material. The loaded tray is rotated in to the oral cavity and all the border molding movements are repeated. Once the material sets, the tray is removed and the impression is inspected. The thin impression paste at the periphery indicates that the border material has compressed the vestibular tissues recording the sulcus in function **(Fig. 3.2.29)**. Therefore, this is also known as a wash impression. There should not be any porosities or discrepancies on the impression surface.

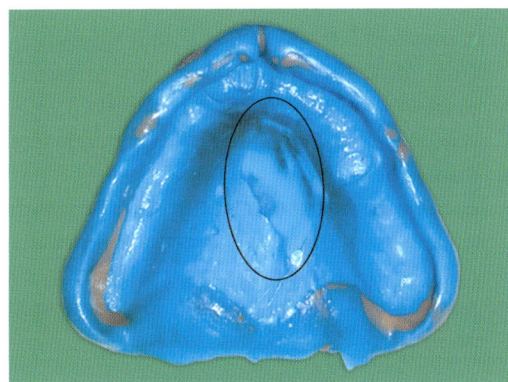

Fig. 3.2.28: Bubble formation in the final impression due to lack of adequate vents

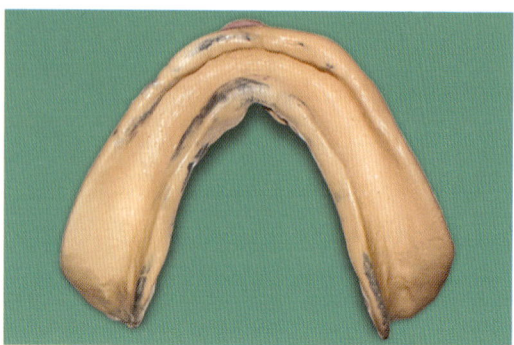

Fig. 3.2.29: Good mandibular final impression showing thin ZOE material over the borders recording sulcus in function

A satisfactory impression is first disinfected as discussed in chapter 3.1, before sending it to the laboratory.

## Beading and Boxing

Beading and boxing are standard procedures to ascertain that all the relevant details from the impression are transferred to the stone cast providing an adequate peripheral border and the land area/protective rim around the cast. Beading protects and preserves the width and height of the recorded sulcus in the cast whereas boxing encloses or boxes the impression to get an adequate sized base.

It is recommended to pour the impression with the help of a vibrating machine as it will lead to reduced porosity/air bubbles. The heavier particles of the stone will also settle at the bottom ie: the top layer of the cast will have the denser particles making the impression surface of the cast stronger and resistant to abrasion.

There are various methods of beading and boxing. The most common method is described below:
- A marker is used to place a line 3 mm below the peripheral roll all around the impression border to discern the extensions
- Place the beaded wax at the marked line. The wax is sticky in nature so easily adapts and adheres to the impression (ZOE impressions)
- For elastomeric silicon impressions the wax does not stick properly therefore, it is recommended to place commercial adhesive at the line before placing the beading wax. Once the bead is stable the edges of the wax can be melted by heating with an instrument to enhance the grip

## Step 3.2 Final Impressions

- The beading wax is placed perpendicular to our impression and must follow the borders below the height of contour
- Boxing wax is placed around the bead and the junction softened to adhere more firmly
- Once the box is ready, the impression is set to be poured with high strength dental stone
- Completed master casts require none to minimal trimming as they are preshaped with beading and boxing.

## Conclusion

- The type and features required in the spacer and the custom tray must be decided by the clinician and prescribed to the technician. Not the other way around.
- The material and technique in final impression making depends on the type of tissues (hard and soft) to be recorded. As tissue quality varies in patients, one method or technique can not be used in all cases.
- Movements done during border molding follow the attachment of muscles in the area and therefore have a specific direction which needs to be respected and followed.

# Step 4

## Registration of Maxillo Mandibular Relations

*"The patient's maxilla-mandibular relationships are dynamic and change during life"*
  Sheldon Winkler

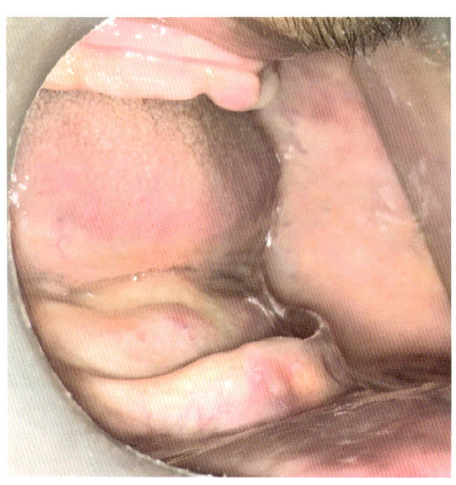

# Step 4

# Registration of Maxillo Mandibular Relations

## ■ INTRODUCTION

There are three relations of maxilla to the mandible which are recorded for complete denture fabrication:
1. Orientation Relation
2. Vertical Dimension
3. Centric Relation.

All three are important but the centric relation has been the most confusing and controversial relation to define and implement in complete denture fabrication. There are more than 26 definitions to explain the centric and these have been changed and modified according to our understanding of anatomy.

Most acceptable definition has been given by Ash which describes how this maxilla mandibular relation is determined clinically. "A maxilla to mandible relationship in which the condyles and disks are thought to be in the midmost, uppermost position **(Fig. 4.1)**. The

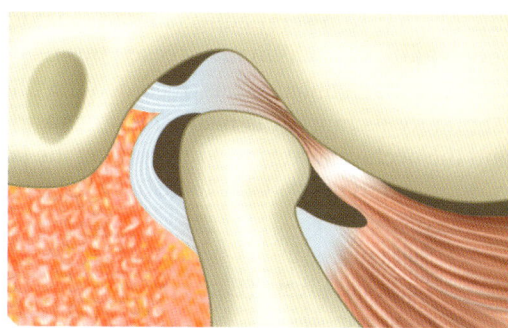

**Fig. 4.1:** The condyle disk assembly

position has been difficult to define anatomically but is determined clinically by assessing when the jaw can hinge on a fixed terminal axis (up to 25 mm). It is a clinically determined relationship of the mandible to the maxilla when the condyle disk assemblies are positioned in their most superior position in the mandibular fossa and against the distal slope of the articular eminence".

Clinically relevant definition according to Dawson, "A properly aligned condyle disc assembly in centric relation can resist maximum loading by the elevator muscles with no signs of discomfort". Centric occlusion is the tooth relation present when the jaws are in centric relation.

Vertical dimension is considered at two levels:
1. Vertical at rest position
2. Vertical at occlusion.

According to GPT8, vertical dimension is defined as: "The distance between two selected anatomic and marked points (usually one on the tip of the nose and the other upon the chin) one on a fixed and one on the movable member".

Though this is a widely accepted definition, one must understand that VDR is a physiological position, the VDO reflects a position chosen by the clinician after assessing all the clinically derived information and is subject to patient and doctor preferences and choices. This relation is subject to change with time as the anatomic points, temporo mandibular joint and denture bearing areas used for assessing vertical dimension have potential for continuous change making jaw relations dynamic in nature.

The scope of achieving the orientation relation, which in simple terms is the orientation of the maxilla to the TMJ is limited as it can only be achieved by using a face bow **(Fig. 4.2)** which can transfer this relation to a semi adjustable articulator **(Fig. 4.3)**. If using a simpler articulator as in many cases, this relation is not accessible.

Once the clinician has recorded the final impressions, the laboratory technician is instructed to construct the denture bases and the occlusal wax rims for recording the jaw relations. There are various materials available to be used as denture bases such as:
- Acrylic resin:
    - Self cure resin
    - Light cure resin **(Figs 4.4 and 4.5)**
    - Heat cure resin.

## Step 4  Registration of Maxillo Mandibular Relations

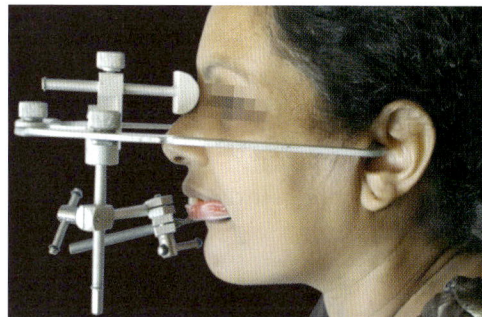

Fig. 4.2: Orientation of the maxilla to the mandible achieved using a facebow

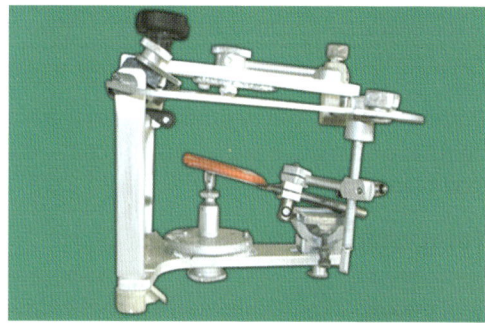

Fig. 4.3: Orientation relation transferred to a semi adjustable articulator

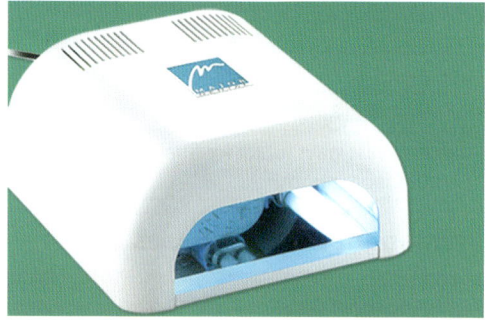

Fig. 4.4: Light curing machine having ultraviolet tubes for curing

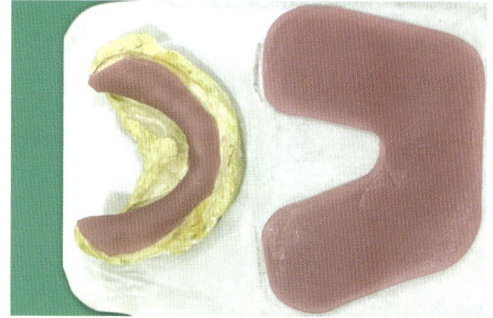

Fig. 4.5: Light cured denture base material and adapted mandibular base

- Base metal alloy
- Shellac base plate: Thermoplastic
- Wax.

These materials can also be classified according to their incorporation in the final dentures **(Table 4.1)**.

Table 4.1: **Denture base classification**

| Temporary Denture Bases | Permanent Denture Base |
|---|---|
| Thermoplastic materials: Shellac | Non precious metal alloy: Base metal |
| Self cured and light cured acrylic resin | Heat cured acrylic resin |
| Wax | |

Both temporary and definitive denture bases are utilized by various dentists on a regular basis and both have their set of advantages and disadvantages.

## Temporary Denture Bases

| Advantages | Disadvantages |
|---|---|
| Ease of manipulation construction | Less stable in the mouth especially if resorbed ridge is present |
| Cheaper | Less rigid |
| Less time consuming | Difficult to use during jaw relation |
| Working cast stays intact for final denture fabrication | Inferior adaptation to the underlying tissues |

## Permanent Denture Bases

| Advantages | Disadvantages |
|---|---|
| Superior tissue adaptation | Working cast is destroyed |
| Dimensionally very stable | Expensive |
| Extremely rigid | Acrylic is subject to an additional curing cycle which theoretically may lead to warpage of the base |
| Ease and accuracy during jaw relation | Technical and time consuming fabrication |

**Step 4** Registration of Maxillo Mandibular Relations

## Fabrication of Permanent Denture Base

Procedure for inclusion of the permanent denture bases into the final dentures:-

As the final impressions are poured, the stone working cast is obtained by cast duplication. The waxed up base is placed onto the cast and it is flasked, dewaxed, processed, deflasked and polished. Metal denture bases are used in patients with a history of midline(palatal) denture fractures and bruxism. Their selection should be made keeping in mind that they are heavier and are difficult to adjust as compared to heat cured acrylic bases. Newer high impact alternatives are also available these days.

## Occlusal Wax Rim Fabrication

Modeling wax is utilized to fabricate rims on the denture bases. Wax is heated and placed in the form of the underlying arch form. For maxilla it is usually a horse shoe shape and for mandible it is a wide "U" shape following the arch form **(Fig. 4.6)**.

### *Maxillary Occlusal Wax Rim*

Many factors contribute to the height of the rim:
- The lip length
- Lip fullness
- Tooth visibility: Patient's choice.

Though, the rim has to be adjusted in the patient's mouth by the dentist, the reductions and additions are a tedious process. Using a scale or a papillometer, just under the lip near the labial frenum helps in determining the approximate height of the wax rim which

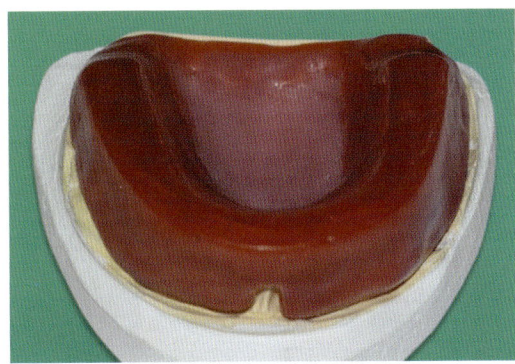

Fig. 4.6: Horse shoe shaped maxillary wax rim

can then be conveyed to the technician. This helps in getting the correct height of the maxillary rim saving chair time.

Other important factors:
- Orientation of the rim:
  - Interpupillary line parallelism to the anterior wax rim
  - Ala tragus line parallel to the posterior rim forming the curve of spee **(Fig. 4.7)**. Confirmed with the help of fox plane or assessed by a thorough visual examination.
- Naso labial angle: Approximately 90 degrees to check the labial profile of the patient **(Fig. 4.8)**.

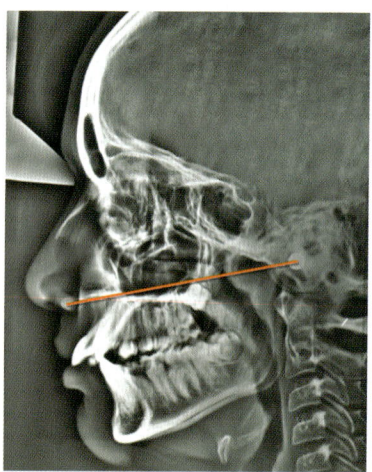

**Fig. 4.7:** A line drawn through Ala tragus is parallel to the posterior teeth (Posterior occlusal rim in denture patients) forming the curve of spee

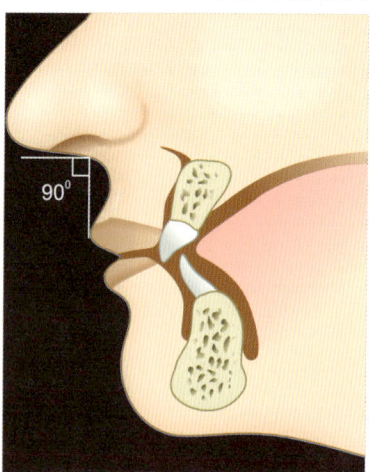

**Fig. 4.8:** Nasolabial angle: 90 degrees

### Step 4 Registration of Maxillo Mandibular Relations

#### *Mandibular Wax Rim*

Reference points **(Fig. 4.9)**:
- Posteriorly, the wax rim should be placed on the center of the ridge. This ensures that the fossa of the mandibular denture teeth lie on a line bisecting the width of the mandibular rim
- The height of the rim should intersect the retromolar pad at 2/3rd or half level. It is subject to alteration in the oral cavity. The occlusal plane thus formed is important as a high plane will cause difficulty in mastication and food bolus placement on the teeth where as a low plane will result in cheek bite
- Anterior rim should be at the level of the vermilion border and flush with the level of the modiolus at the corner of the mouth
- With age the visibility of the mandibular teeth increases, thus the height of the rim may be kept in the visibility range of 0.5-1.5 mm
- Lingual contour of the wax rim should be concave with a slight gingival roll to it. This allows the tongue to settle/sit partially there. Advantages: Prevention of tongue bite and stability of the lower denture as the tongue keeps it in place **(Fig. 4.10)**.

## Determination of the Vertical Dimension

Various methods used are:
- Rest position (Vertical Dimension ot Rest) **(Fig. 4.11)**:
    - Freeway space of 2-4 mm in the first premolar region
    - Asking patient to swallow, relax lower jaw, part lips to view space between the teeth.
- Phonetics: "s" sounds to evaluate average speaking space
- Esthetics and phonetics

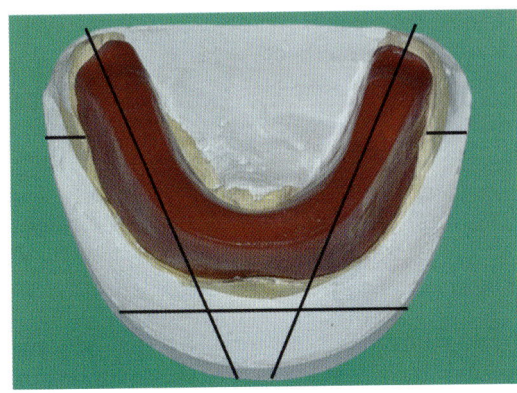

**Fig. 4.9:** Mandibular wax rim: Teeth should be placed on the center of the ridge to enhance stability

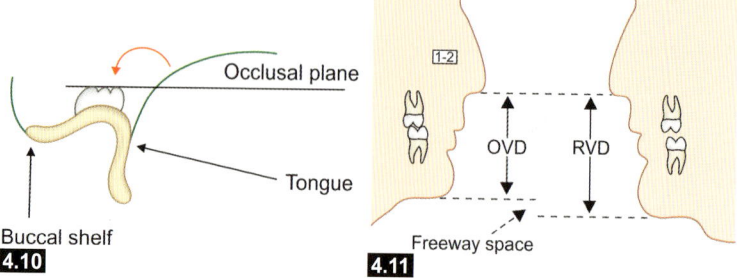

Fig. 4.10: Space for the tongue to settle in.    Fig. 4.11: Freeway space of 2-4 mm

- Swallowing threshold.
- Tactile sense and patient perceived comfort:
  - Neuromuscular perception.
- Facial parameters for VDO versus VDR with dots on face, specifically using landmarks such as chin to nose distance-Niswonger's method **(Fig. 4.12)**.

One and all methods are used in combination to determine the vertical dimension. The amount of free way space can be checked with a measuring gauge or a divider and still remains the principal method of recording the vertical dimension **(Fig. 4.13)**.

Signs and symptoms of excessive increase and decrease in vertical dimension (VD) are mentioned in **Table 4.2**.

Table 4.2: Excessive increase and decrease in VD

| Excessive Increase in VD | Excessive Decrease in VD |
|---|---|
| Clicking sound as teeth touch sooner than intended | Inefficiency: Masticatory ability is hampered |
| Trauma: Temporomandibular joints, mucosa, underlying bone | Cheek biting |
| Enhanced bone resorption | Pain in temporomandibular joints |
| Swallowing difficulty | Dribbling of saliva from the corners of the mouth |
| Long face: Elongation of face **(Fig. 4.14)** | Older senile appearance with smaller looking face and deeper line angles **(Fig. 4.15)** |
| Dry mouth: Lips parted all the time | Angular chelitis |

When adjustments are complete, the wax rims are ready for centric relation record. There are various methods that have been used in

## Step 4  Registration of Maxillo Mandibular Relations

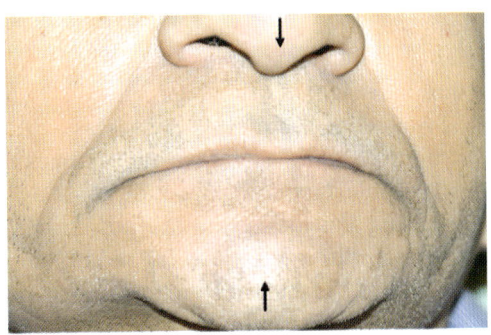

**Fig. 4.12:** Facial support for Vertical Dimension at Occlusion versus Vertical dimension at rest measured with dots/reference points on the face

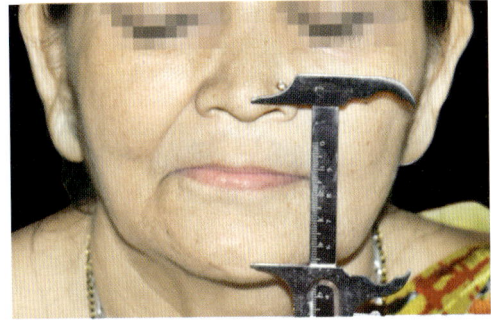

**Fig. 4.13:** A Caliper is used to measure, record and lock the vertical dimension

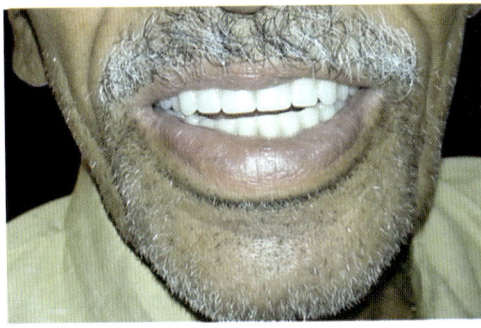

**Fig. 4.14:** Long face syndrome: elongation of face due to increased vertical dimension in the complete dentures

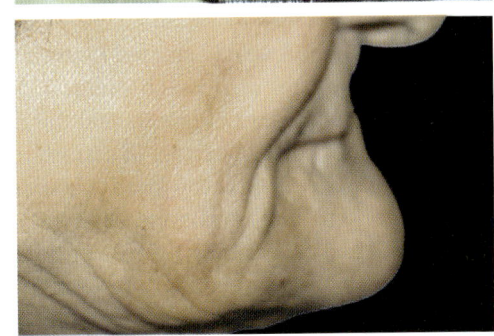

**Fig. 4.15:** Smaller looking face with wrinkled appearance due to decreased vertical dimension

the past and are still relevant when it comes to recording the centric relation. Clinicians still use the following methods to retrude the mandible in a comfortable, repeatable position:
- Swallowing method: Patient is asked to swallow and close the mouth. As the mandible moves back the condyle comes in a favorable, recordable position
- Placing the tongue on the posterior aspect of the palate and taking it further back as the mouth closes. Disadvantage of this technique is that there are chances of over retrusion
- Dawson's Bimanual manipulation: This method though used commonly in dentate patients, helps to achieve centric relation with ease even in edentulous patients.

Procedure: **(Fig. 4.16)**:
- **Step 1:** Recline the patient all the way back in a supine position
- **Step 2:** Stabilize the head level. Top of the patient's head in center of the abdomen, cradle the head between the ribcage and the forearm.
  - Lift the patient's chin up, to slightly stretch the neck
  - Position the four fingers of each hand on the lower border of the mandible
  - Bring the thumbs together to form a "C" with each hand
  - Gently manipulate the jaw so it slowly hinges open and closed: It will slip in to centric if no pressure is applied.

Once the patient goes into centric without difficulty, the clinician must check the position and make the patient repeat it before locking the rims in place. The material used most commonly to record and lock the rims in centric relation is Aluwax. Some clinicians prefer to use hard, silicon bite registration materials for ease of workability and to do away with hot water manipulation which is required to soften the wax.

**Creation of Seal:** A seal is created between the two rims at centric relation by the Nick and notch method. Many clinicians use hot instruments such as wax knife to seal the rims **(Fig. 4.17)**, it is not the method of choice. Chances of distortion, movement and errors in orientation are some of the disadvantages of this technique. Once the rims are sealed there is no way to check the centric again in the mouth which is considered a major disadvantage. Score marks are placed on the rims to ensure correct reassembling if the rims get separated.

## Step 4 Registration of Maxillo Mandibular Relations

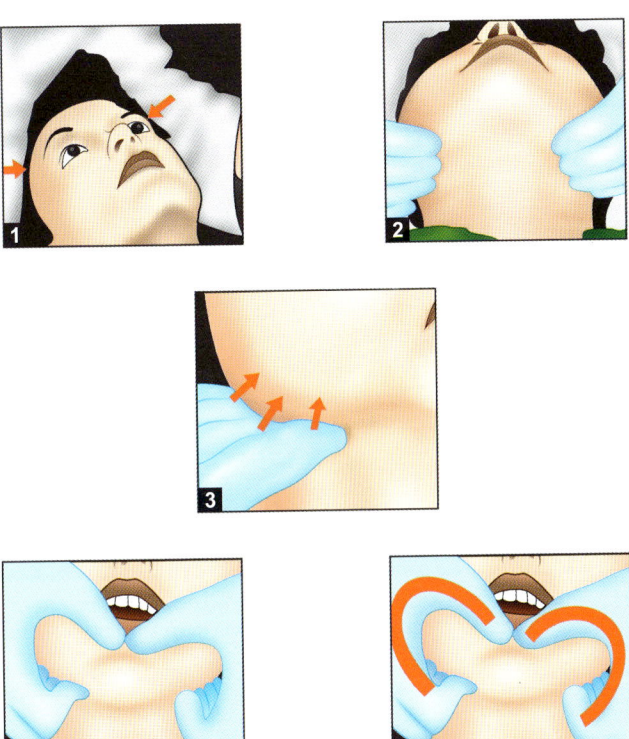

Fig. 4.16: Dawsons Method of Bimannual manipulation; Step 1: Stabilize the head. Step 2: After the head is stabilized, lift patient's chin again to slightly stretch the neck. Step 3: Gently position four fingers of each hand on the lower border of the mandible. Step 4A and B: Bring thumbs together to form a C with each hand

**Nick and Notch method:** The most accepted procedure. **(Figs 4.18 to 4.20)**
- Cut a trough of 3-4mm on the mandibular wax rim, ending just before the most mesial part **(Fig. 4.21A)**
- Nick and notch are created in the maxillary occlusal rim on the area corresponding the trough **(Fig. 4.21B)**
- Both nick and notch have the distal slope at 90 degrees to stop the flow of bite registration material further, where as the distal slope is at an angle to allow the material to fill the space
- Bite registration material is placed and the mandible is manipulated into centric as the patient closes the mouth

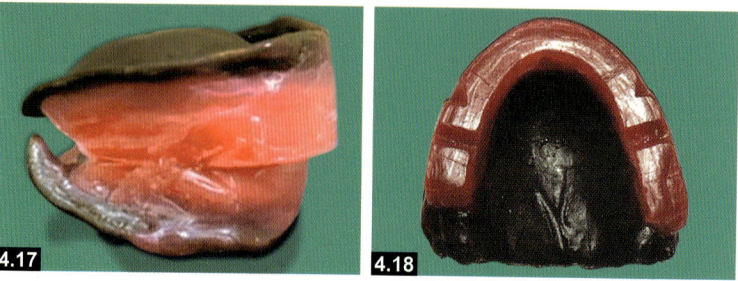

**Fig. 4.17:** Most commonly used method: Hot instrument to seal the wax rims.
**Fig. 4.18:** Nick and notch method for recording the centric relation

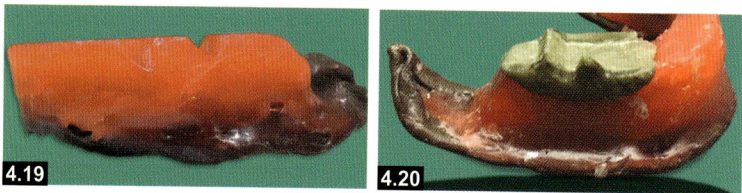

**Fig. 4.19:** Nick and notch created in the maxillary wax rim.
**Fig. 4.20:** Nick and notch replicated with Aluwax in the mandibular denture

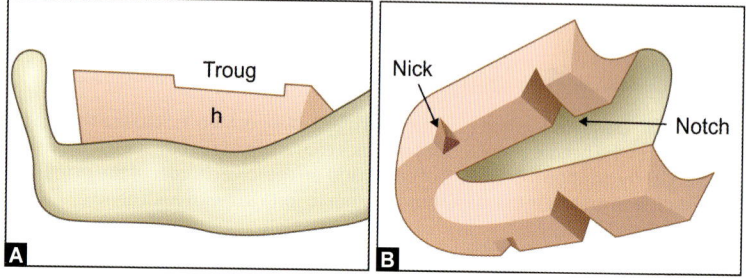

**Figs 4.21A and B:** Nick and notch method graphical representation

- Once the occlusal rims are flush against each other, the material is allowed to set
- Remove and cut excess material
- Open and place the rims again in the mouth and recheck the centric relation. It should fit perfectly.

Graphic Methods: These are used in case of facebow transfer and mounting on a semi adjustable articulator. Interocclusal records are made as arrow point tracing is achieved with a gothic arch tracer **(Figs 4.22, 4.23A and B, 4.24)**.

## Step 4 Registration of Maxillo Mandibular Relations

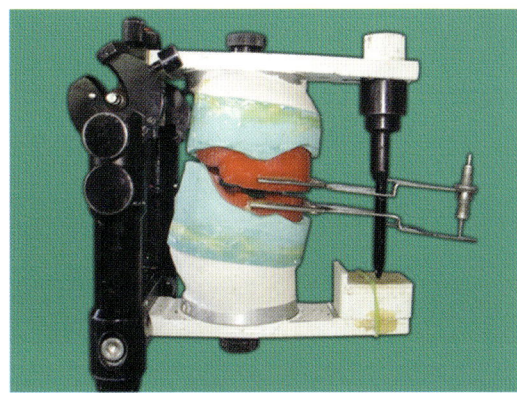

Fig. 4.22: Extra oral tracers

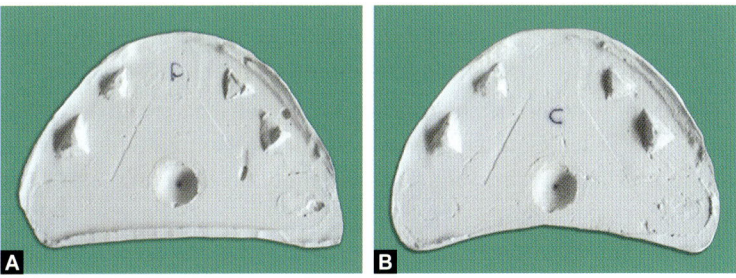

Figs 4.23A and B: (A) Interocclusal protrusive record. (B) Interocclusal centric record. Both made in plaster of paris

Types:
- Intra-oral
- Extra-oral.

Arrow tracing is formed by making the patient do centric and eccentric movements: Protrusive, right lateral and left lateral. It is repeatable and the same tracing can be achieved every single time.

Long term studies prove that in most edentulous patients, a mean value articulator produces acceptable results. The use of bilateral balanced occlusion in comparison to the basic maximum intercuspation at centric shows slight difference in chewing efficiency but the difference is not statistically relevant.

Articulators used in complete denture fabrication:
- Hinge type articulator: Allows only vertical movement
- 3 point/mean value articulator: Most commonly used

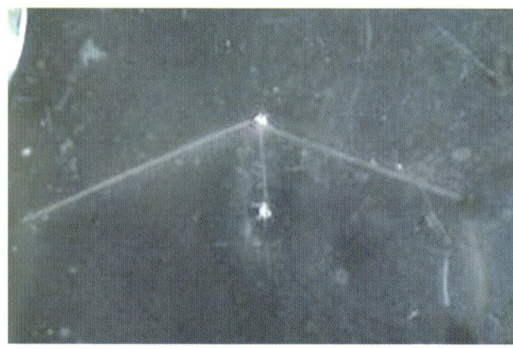

Fig 4.24: Arrow shaped Gothic arch tracing

- Semi adjustable articulator: Allows horizontal and vertical movements, simulating condylar pathways for movements
- Fully adjustable articulator: Allows 3 dimentional dynamic registrations. Rarely used in complete denture construction.

Semi adjustable articulators are used when a balanced occlusion is desired. A facebow transfer is done first to simulate the relation of the maxillary arch to the TMJ assembly on the articulator **(Fig. 4.25)**.

Once the maxillary cast is mounted in the correct orientation, the rims are sealed in centric in the patient's mouth and the lower cast is also mounted keeping the centric intact.

As the plaster is set, the rims can be separated and the technician can proceed with teeth arrangement.

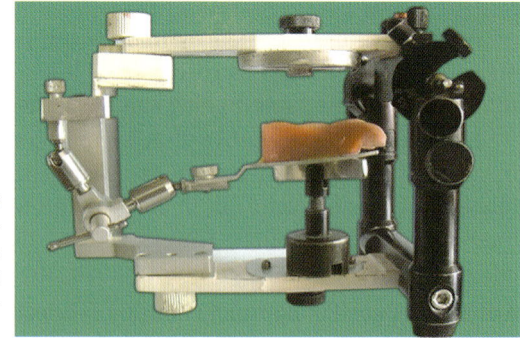

Fig. 4.25: A facebow transfer is done to simulate the relation of the maxillary cast to the TMJ assembly on the articulator

## Step 4 Registration of Maxillo Mandibular Relations

## Tips and Tricks

- Permanent bases especially the heat cure acrylic and the temporary cold cure acrylic bases are stable and make the task of recording jaw relation easy, in comparison to the shellac base plate material
- Occlusal rims adjustment must follow a step by step protocol:
  - Shape the maxillary rim according to the esthetic requirements utilizing the said landmarks
  - Mandibular wax rim is adjusted after the maxillary rim is shaped to achieve the correct vertical
- Always give space for the buccal corridor as this negative space must be created during manipulation of the wax rims. It gives the illusion of depth and beauty
- While recording the vertical, if one can't be exact it is preferable to have slightly reduced vertical than an excessive vertical dimension for patient comfort
- One must never use force ie: push/pull the mandible to achieve centric relation as the jaw gets pushed to the most retruded position rather than the desired one
- In my limited experience Dawson's Bimanual manipulation gives most acceptable and reproducible results while recording centric relation
- Always ascertain that while recording the centric relation, the denture bases do not touch posteriorly as that can lead to a shift in the mandible leading to wrong centric **(Fig. 4.26)**.

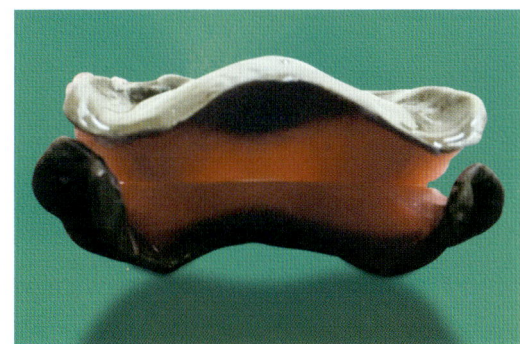

Fig. 4.26: Ensure that the denture bases do not touch posteriorly post centric relation

## Conclusion

- Centric relation is the only clinically reproducible and repeatable jaw position in complete denture prosthesis fabrication.
- Centric occlusion / Maximum intercuspation in complete denture patients should coincide with centric relation position.
- Long term studies prove that in most edentulous patients, a mean value articulator produces acceptable results. The use of bilateral balanced occlusion in comparison to the basic maximum intercuspation at centric shows slight difference in chewing efficiency but the difference is not statistically relevant.

# Step 5

## Anterior Try in Aesthetic Considerations

*"What the thought is to the word,
the feeling is to the facial expression"*
*Scottish physiologist Charles bell (1774-1842)*

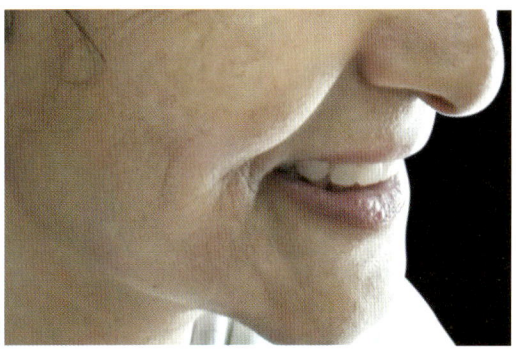

# Step 5

# Anterior Try in Aesthetic Considerations

## ■ INTRODUCTION

Denture esthetics is a complex process of understanding the edentulous hard and soft tissues, along with the clinician's dexterity to choose and place the best suited materials giving a natural appearance. Each patient is unique and so is his or her denture. A clinician must respect that and strive to deliver dentures which match individual patient's character and appearance.

Post extraction bone resorption, i.e. centripetal resorption is seen in maxillary arch leading to a smaller looking maxilla as the buccal bone is more prone to resorption here with reduced lip support **(Fig. 5.1)**. Mandible shows increased bone loss at the lingual side compared to buccal forming a wide "V" resulting in a centrifugal type of resorption **(Fig. 5.2)**. This sometimes complicates the teeth selection and arrangement process. Therefore, a thorough understanding of

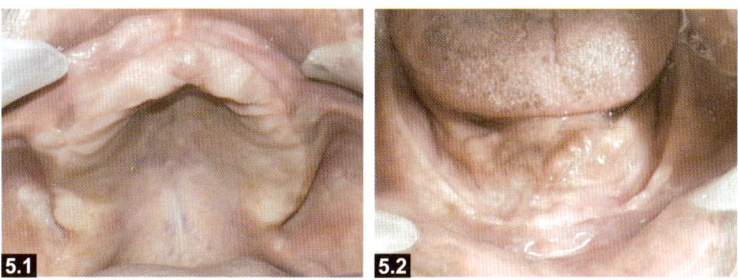

Fig. 5.1: Centripetal resorption leading to small maxilla. Fig. 5.2: Centrifugal type of resorption leading to V shaped mandibular arch

the biological and physiological process is needed to determine and explain to the patient the realistic esthetic possibilities.

Biometric guides utilizing epithelial bands (gingival margin bands) and anthropometric measurements have been used time and again to determine the ideal placement of denture teeth and to simulate preextraction tooth positioning.

Some of the old school methods are as follows:

1. Width of maxillary CI = $\dfrac{\text{Circumference of the head}}{13}$

2. Total width of maxillary anteriors = $\dfrac{\text{Bizygomatic width}}{3.36}$

3. Width of the maxillary CI = $\dfrac{\text{Zygomatic width}}{16}$

Determining the tooth size or placement with these guides is not only cumbersome but also not effective. It has been observed that teeth selected by such guides may not be acceptable by the patient as they simulate the size and positioning of a dentate patient.

The changes in the hard and soft tissue anatomy after tooth loss are profound making these measurements inappropriate for tooth selection and their use questionable.

## ▪ DYNESTHETIC OR DENTOGENIC CONCEPT

Denture aesthetics is not a single step consideration, but it starts as soon as the patient walks in the operatory. The concept of relating tooth form to extraoral factors such as facial form and pattern, age were proposed long back in 1950s. Frush and Fisher came up with the sex, personality and age (SPA) factors for teeth selection and characterization **(Table 5.1)**.

Visualizing the esthetic outcome and then translating it to a satisfactory final realistic patient specific result is what the clinician should aim for in complete denture esthetics.

There are various methodologies as mentioned earlier but one needs to choose patient specific methods only as a guide, as the final esthetic scheme must be unique to the patient.

## Step 5  Anterior Try in Aesthetic Considerations

**Table 5.1:** Sex, personality and age (SPA) factors for teeth selection and characterization

| S | Sex | Females | Males |
|---|---|---|---|
|   |   | Rounded teeth<br>Smaller laterals<br>Labioversion (laterals higher, overlapping the centrals) **(Fig. 5.3)** | Sharper teeth<br>Larger laterals<br>Linguoversion (centrals overlapping the laterals) |
| P | Personality | *Vigorous* | *Delicate* |
|   |   | Wider central incisors<br>Sharp line and point angles **(Fig. 5.4A)**<br>Darker shade<br>Wearing of incisor<br>Squarish incisors | Paler teeth<br>Rounded tooth margins<br>Lateral: neck tucked in<br>Small and sharp canines<br>Rounded arch form<br>**(Fig. 5.4B)** |
| A | Age | *Appearance of Youth* | *Older Appearance* |
|   |   | Maxillary teeth more visible<br>Anteriors closely follow the lower lip: smile arc<br>Lighter shade<br>Translucency in the incisal third<br>**(Fig. 5.4C)** | Wearing of incisors<br>Proximal wear<br>Lower teeth more visible<br>Cervical portion more visible and prominent<br>Stains and darker shade<br>**(Fig. 5.4D)** |

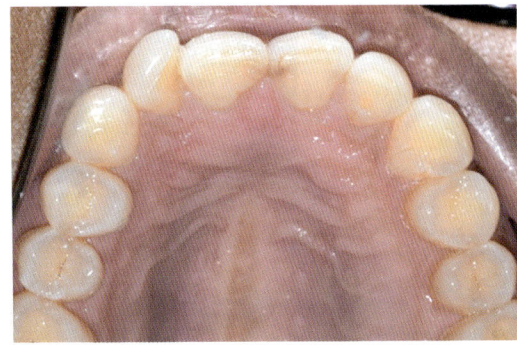

**Fig 5.3:** Labioversion of the lateral incisor, overlapping the central is a very common female characteristic

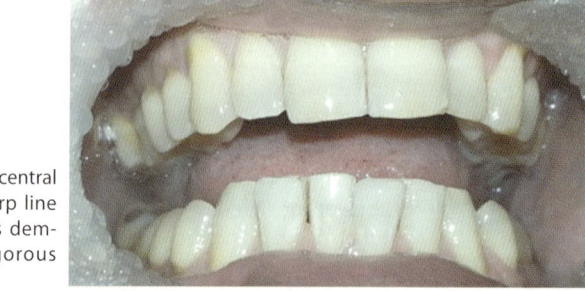

**Fig. 5.4A:** Wide central incisors with sharp line and point angles demonstrating a vigorous personality

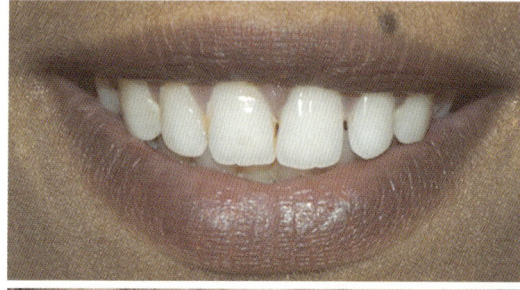

**Fig. 5.4B:** Rounded, pale, small teeth in a round arch form showcase a delicate personality

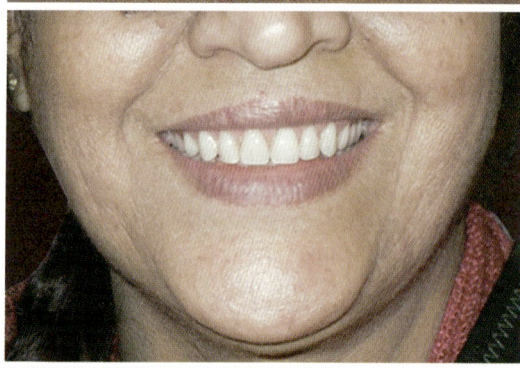

**Fig. 5.4C:** Appearance of youth

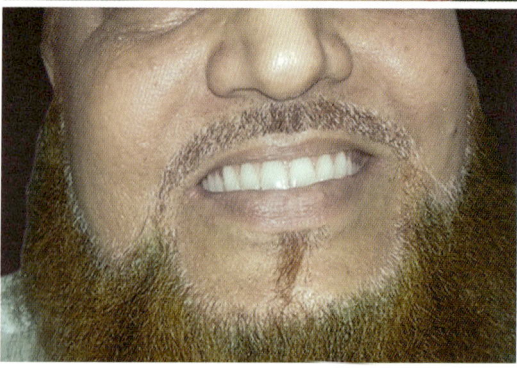

**Fig. 5.4D:** Older appearance exaggerated by using teeth with dark shade and wearing of incisors

**Step 5** Anterior Try in Aesthetic Considerations

## Preextraction Guides

- Diagnostic casts: Patient's preextraction models
- Photographs: Preextraction pictures
- Radiographs: Teeth shape can be determined but size is usually enlarged so can't be used as a criteria.

## Postextraction Examination

- Size and shape of the residual alveolar ridges
- Ridge relation **(Fig. 5.5)**
- Lip thickness
- Lip length
- Arch form
- Facial frontal form
- Facial profile **(Fig. 5.6)**
- Interarch space **(Fig. 5.7)**
- Intercuspid distance **(Fig. 5.8)**
- Smile line.

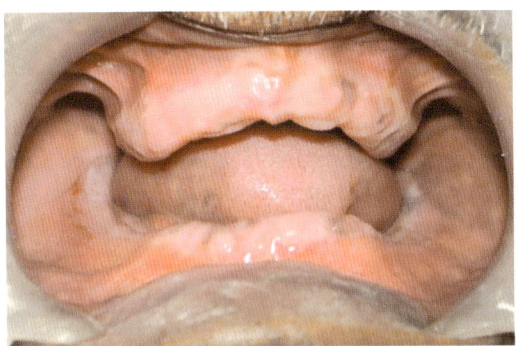

Fig. 5.5: Ideal ridge relation showing healthy maxillary and mandibular denture bearing areas

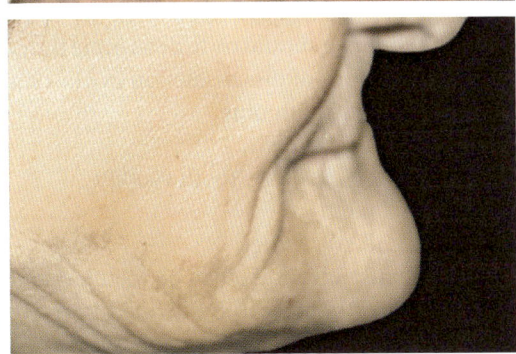

Fig. 5.6: Facial profile of an edentulous patient without denture

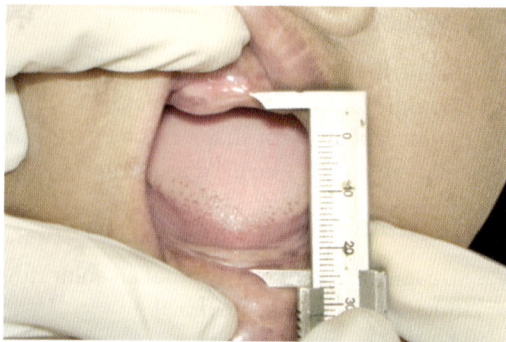

**Fig. 5.7:** Post extraction inter arch space measured at the incisor and the premolar regions

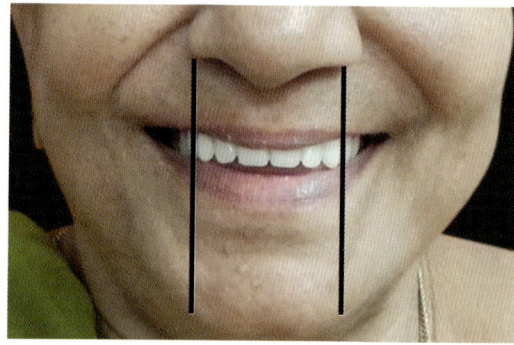

**Fig. 5.8:** Measurement of the intercuspid distance in 2 ways: (1) Measure the distance between the canine eminences. (2) Distance between distal of the canines in existing denture wearers

In old-denture wearers, the clinician should ask the patient for any esthetic complaints and then place the dentures in the oral cavity and assess the old denture esthetics.

If the patient is satisfied functionally and esthetically and the clinician feels that the denture is sound, then old denture tooth mould can be duplicated. As anterior teeth also influence the speech patterns, the familiar shapes and positioning will make things easier.

If the patient is dissatisfied with the old denture's appearance then, the clinician should try to determine the cause of dissatisfaction. Common reasons of dissatisfaction in old-denture wearers:
- Darker shade with time
- Attrited incisor teeth
- Insufficient maxillary tooth visibility
- Chipped teeth
- Stains and crack lines.

Once the cause is found it can be rectified in the new dentures.

Anterior esthetics can be divided into two distinct sections i.e. teeth selection and teeth arrangement.

Step 5 Anterior Try in Aesthetic Considerations

## TEETH SELECTION

It is determined by the following:

### Size of the Tooth

**Length of the tooth determined by:** Smile line, lip line, inter occlusal distance

**Width of the tooth determined by:** Intercanine distance and SPA factors.

### Shape or Form of the Tooth

**Facial form:** Leon William's concept **(Fig. 5.9)**.

**Arch form: (Fig. 5.10)**.

**Profile of the face:** Facial profile is determined by following **(Fig 5.11 A to C and 5.12)**:

- Forehead
- Base of the nose
- Chin, the most prominent part.

The ridge relation, bony prominence and lip support all play an important role in teeth selection and arrangement. The labioincisal contour of the anterior teeth confirms to the profile of the patient and when viewed from the side should be in harmony with the rest of the face **(Fig. 5.13)**.

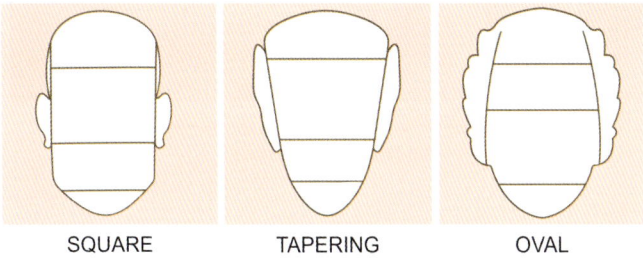

Fig. 5.9: Types of facial form

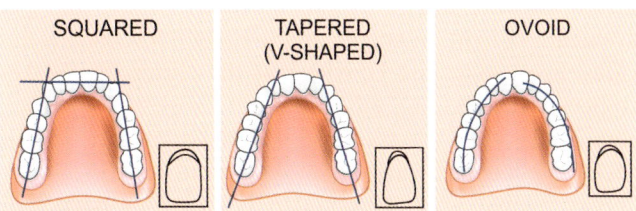

Fig. 5.10: Types of arch form

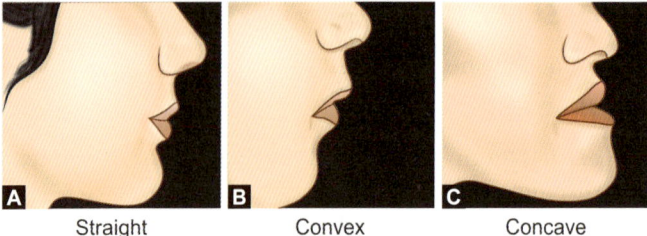

Figs 5.11A to C: Facial profile depending on the chin size and position

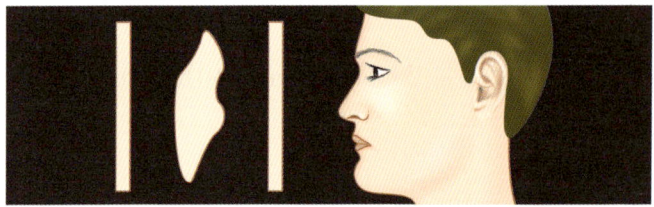

Fig. 5.12: Examination of facial profile

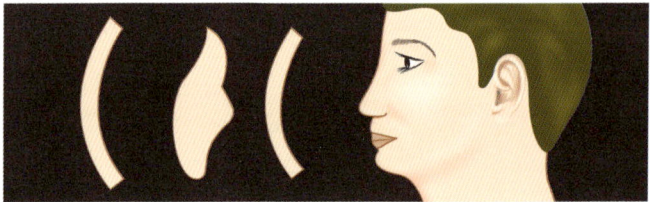

Fig. 5.13: The labio-incisal contour of the anterior teeth confirms to the profile of the patient

## Tooth Color

- **Hue and chroma:** It is the color of the tooth based on the specific wavelength of light. In acrylic denture teeth, it is usually in four shades, i.e. A, B,C, and D, where as the chroma is marked as numbers 1-4, i.e. A1, A2, A3, A4.
- **Value/Brilliance:** It is the lightness or darkness of the teeth. Caucasians, people with lighter skin tone have darker teeth whereas people with darker skin complexion have whiter/brighter teeth with less color saturation.

## Step 5 Anterior Try in Aesthetic Considerations

- **Translucency:** It is the property of the tooth wherein it allows certain amount of passage of light without giving any clear image thus causing translucency in the tooth. Teeth selection therefore must be done under natural lighting or under color corrected lights whenever possible **(Fig. 5.14)**.

Teeth arrangement is based on positioning of the teeth which is determined by many extraoral and intraoral factors.

## Relation of Incisors to the Relevant Planes

The relation of incisors with different types of relevant planes is elaborated in **Table 5.2**.

Table 5.2: Relation of incisors to the relevant planes

| Relevant Plane | Relation of Incisors |
|---|---|
| Midsagittal plane **(Fig. 5.15)** | Central incisor placed at 15–16 degrees from the side profile. |
| | The maxillary wax rim at the time of jaw relation must be adjusted to a 75 degree angulation to the occlusal plane for teeth to be placed at this inclination. |
| Transverse plane **(Fig. 5.16)** | Edge of central incisors touch the occlusal plane whereas lateral incisors are arranged 0.5–1 mm away. |
| | Incisal edges are parallel to the interpupillary line. |
| Frontal plane **(Fig. 5.17)** | Central incisors are placed with a very slight mesial inclination toward the midline whereas lateral incisor's mesial inclination is comparatively more pronounced. |
| | Midline discrepancy if present needs to be corrected at this stage **(Fig. 5.18)** |

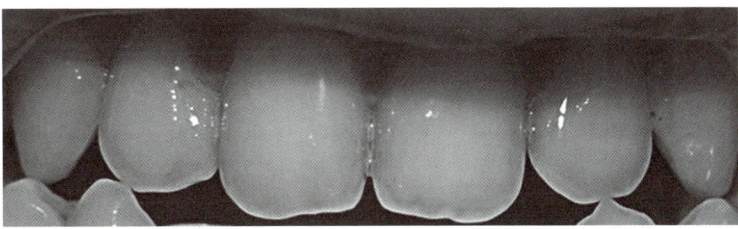

Fig. 5.14: Translucency

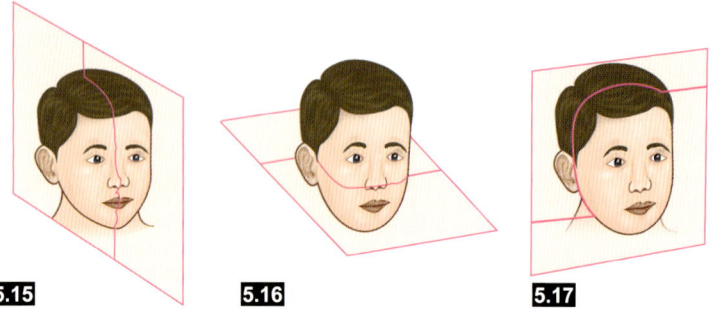

Fig. 5.15: Midsagittal plane.   Fig. 5.16: Transverse plane.   Fig. 5.17: Frontal plane

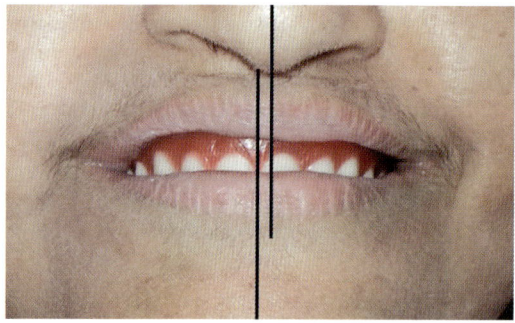

Fig. 5.18: Midline discrepancy between the dental and the facial midline. Studies show that it is acceptable if the discrepancy is with in 4mm of each other. More than 4 mm is noticeable to the patient

## ■ THE GOLDEN PROPORTION

It is a universal proportion based on mathematics and nature. In dentistry, it is one of the many ways suggested for teeth arrangement. It is based on the viewing width, i.e. what is seen rather than the actual width of the teeth.

Following this ratio known as the repeated ration, the central incisors are dominant with laterals and the cuspid (visible portion) becoming progressively smaller. Here, the concept of symmetry and a thorough understanding of the harmony within the orofacial complex is more important than following the exact mathematical proportions **(Figs 5.19 and 5.20)**.

## Buccal Corridor

Buccal corridor is more commonly called the negative space and is seen at the corners of the mouth when the patient is asked to smile. It is a dark space present between the buccal surfaces of the posterior

## Step 5 Anterior Try in Aesthetic Considerations

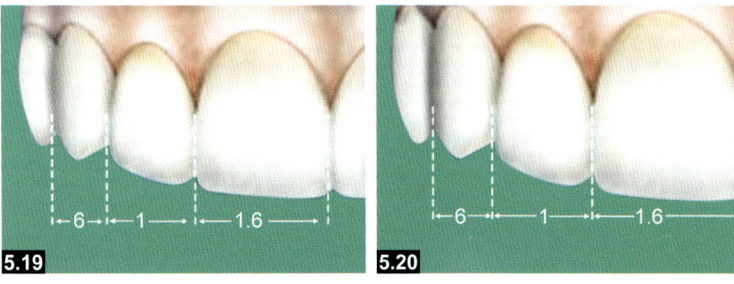

**Fig. 5.19:** Golden proportion with the visible portion of the tooth following the Fibonacci sequence. **Fig. 5.20:** Recurring esthetic dental (RED) proportion or repeated ratio. It means the proportion of the successive width of the teeth remaining constant, when progressing distally from the midline

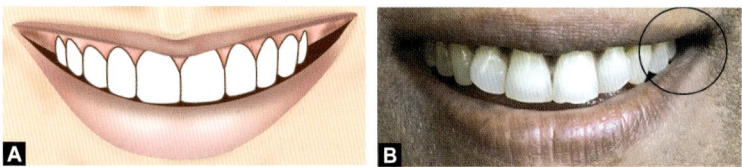

**Figs 5.21A and B:** Buccal corridor: negative space present between the teeth and the buccal mucosa. It is seen as a dark space at the corner of the mouth

teeth (specially the maxillary premolars and the first molar) and the cheek **(Figs 5.21A and B)**.

### Function

Natural appearance by imparting depth to the smile.

### Factors Affecting Buccal Corridor

- Canine prominence
- Maxillary arch:
  - Width
  - Form.
- Facial muscle tone
- Maxillary posterior teeth, specially the premolar and the 1st molar placement.

## ■ DENTURE BASE CHARACTERIZATION

Color matching and contouring of the denture base to simulate gingival oral tissues helps in achieving natural appearance **(Figs 5.22A**

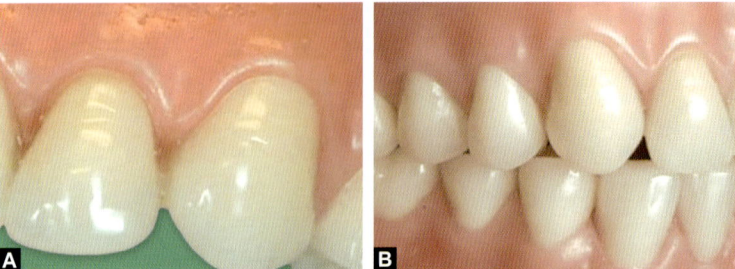

**Figs 5.22A and B:** Contouring of the denture base in wax

**and B)**. Acrylic stains are incorporated within the polymer-monomer during layering prior to packing and acrylization for a more life-like look of the denture base.

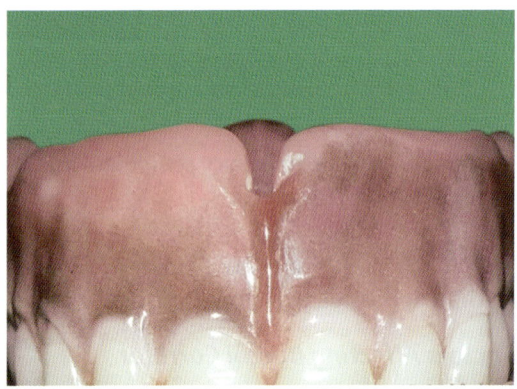

**Fig. 5.23:** Denture base characterization

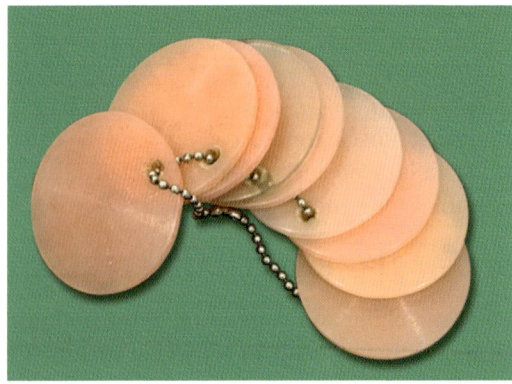

**Fig. 5.24:** Different colors of denture base material

**Step 5** Anterior Try in Aesthetic Considerations

The actual shade and saturation of the tints will vary according to the thickness and color of the acrylic outer layer as usually the colors are incorporated in the deeper layers **(Fig. 5.23 and 5.24)**.

## Recent Advances in Gingival Characterization

Light cure color fluid systems have come in to market which can be applied directly to the outer surface of cured dentures for color characterization in the clinic by the dentist **(Fig. 5.25)**.

## Advantages

- A more personalized denture
- Easy chair-side application and correction
- Smooth finish and polishability.

Compatible with most light curing systems, resulting in more personalized dentures.

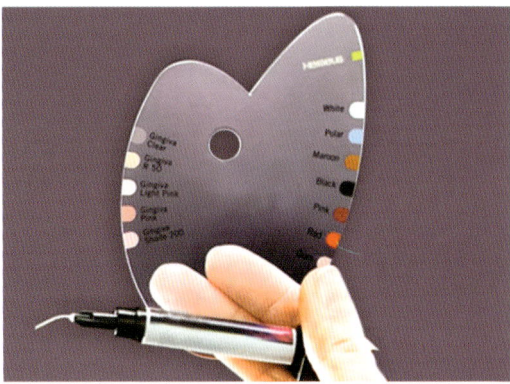

Fig. 5.25: Personalized, chairside color correction system

# Conclusion

- A pleasing appearance not only boosts the confidence of our geriatric patients but many a times is also the difference between success or failure of the prosthesis.
- The patient with the clinician and the clinician with the technician must communicate well to ensure perfect teeth selection and characterization of denture teeth and base.
- The adjusted occlusal rims are an important part of final denture appearance and must be treated so.

# Step 6

## Occlusion

*"Society is made up of happy neurotics, unhappy neurotics, and a few psychotics and some of each become partially or totally edentulous."* (Balance is for parafunctional movements)

Theodore Berg Jr

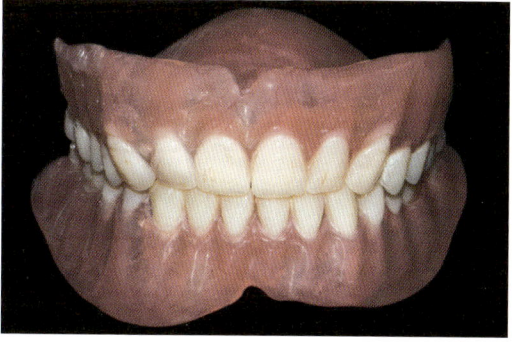

# Step 6

# Occlusion

## INTRODUCTION

Occlusion many a times is used as a synonym to maximum intercuspation which relates to static tooth contacts, where as articulation is a dynamic tooth relationship during centric and eccentric movements.

In this chapter occlusion will imply tooth contacts as static as well as dynamic.

Denture Occlusion being different from natural tooth occlusion requires dealing with many compromising factors:
- Unequal surface areas of maxillary and mandibular arches causing stability issues **(Fig. 6.1)**
- Denture teeth work as a unit and any discrepancy in a single unit can compromise the complete denture occlusion

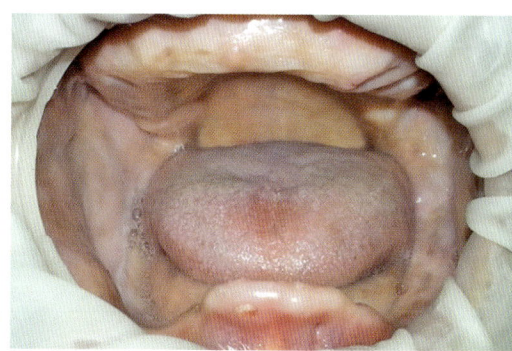

**Fig. 6.1:** Discrepancy in surface areas of maxillary and mandibular arches

- Changes in the denture base area due to continuous, life long bone resorption process **(Fig. 6.2)**.

Due to the various anatomical differences many occlusal schemes have been suggested in the past. There is no clarity as to the evidence suggesting clinical benefits of any one occlusal scheme over another.

Most commonly used concepts in Complete denture occlusion are:
- Bilateral balanced occlusion
- Lingualized occlusion
- Monoplane/Non anatomic occlusion.

All three occlusal schemes strive to enhance denture stability and various tooth anatomy are utilized in these schemes to achieve the most favorable functional results **(Flowchart 6.1, Fig. 6.3)**.

Anatomical and semi anatomical tooth molds are usually used to achieve bilateral balanced occlusion where as flat anatomical tooth molds are utilized for monoplane occlusion.

Lingualized occlusal scheme can be made with the combinations of upper anatomical/semi anatomical tooth molds along with a lower non anatomic/flat tooth mold. Many companies have launched newer lingualized molds to facilitate this occlusal scheme.

Therefore, teeth with lingualized features are also added to the regular tooth anatomy **(Figs 6.4 and 6.5)**.

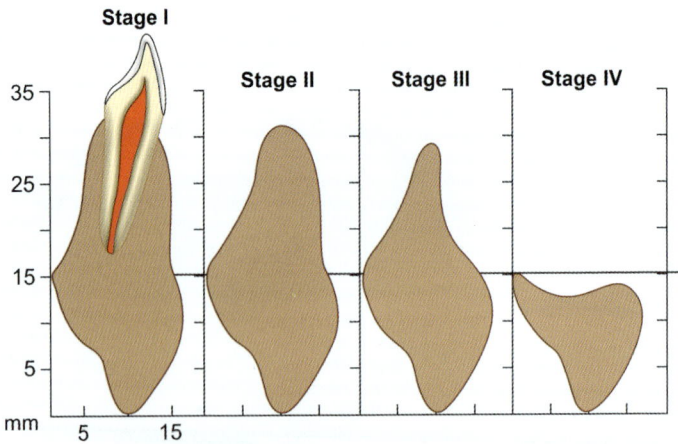

Fig. 6.2: Changes in the denture base area

## Step 6 Occlusion

**Flowchart 6.1:** Types of tooth anatomy

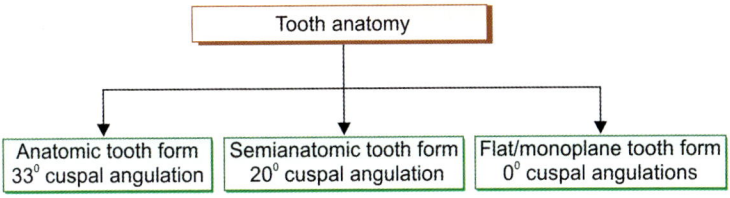

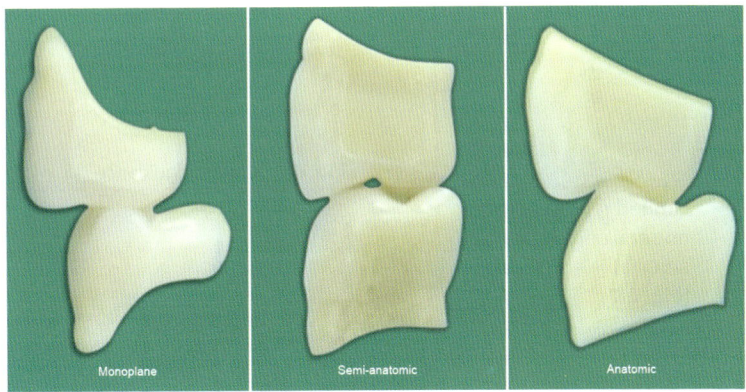

**Fig. 6.3:** Occlusal schemes

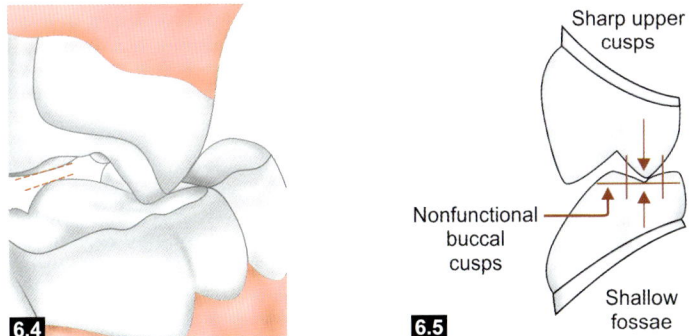

**Figs 6.4 and 6.5:** Lingualized molds to facilitate lingual occlusal scheme. Lingualized occlusal scheme

## HANAU'S QUINT

In complete denture construction, four factors out of the five are in clinician's hands.

| Condylar guidance cannot be altered by the dentist | |
|---|---|
| • Related to the condylar movement in the glenoid fossa during excursive movements **(Fig. 6.6)** | 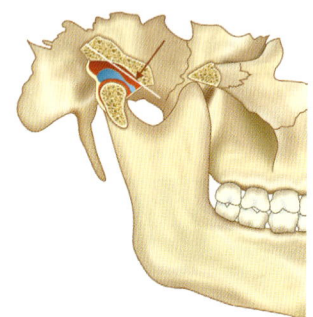<br>Fig. 6.6: Condylar guidance |
| • Limited representation on semi adjustable/fully adjustable articulators **(Fig. 6.7)** | 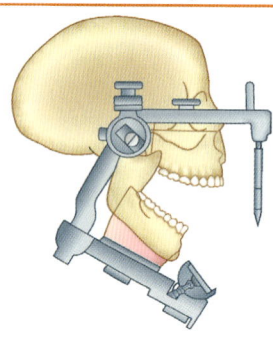<br>Fig. 6.7: Arcon articulator |
| **Incisal guidance determined by dentist** | |
| • Zero degrees is preferred but due to cosmetic reasons minimal i.e: greater than zero is required **(Fig. 6.8)**<br>• Reduces tipping/lateral forces enhancing denture stability | 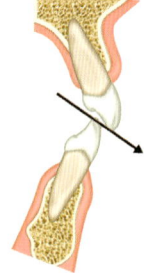<br>Fig. 6.8: Minimal Incisal guidance |

## Step 6  Occlusion

### Plane of occlusion

- Determined by external reference marks such as inter pupillary line and ala-tragus line **(Fig. 6.9)**

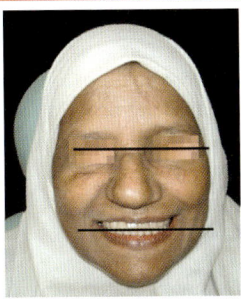

Fig. 6.9: Plane of occlusion parallel to the interpupillary line

- Wax rims during jaw relation stage determine the occlusal plane.
- Incorrect plane may result in canting causing functional instability interferences and compromised esthetic results **(Figs 6.10A and B)**

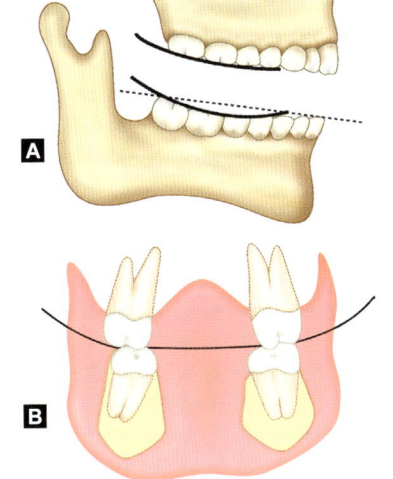

Figs 6.10A and B: Curve of Spee and Wilson

### Cuspal inclination/height

- Cusp slopes or inclinations determine cusp angles **(Fig. 6.11)**
- These are used according to the occlusal scheme, denture base area and desired functional efficiency and esthetic requirement

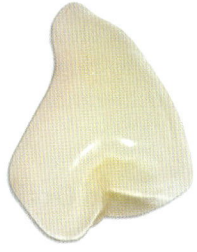

Fig. 6.11: Cuspal inclination

### Compensating curves

Compensatory curves are introduced in denture occlusion for maintaining balance and articulation **(Figs 6.12 and 6.13)**

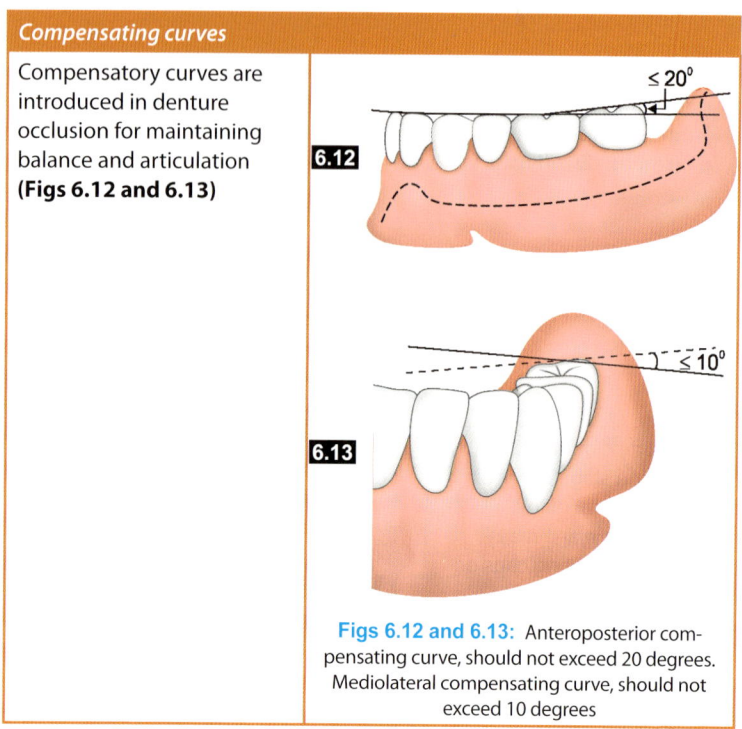

**Figs 6.12 and 6.13:** Anteroposterior compensating curve, should not exceed 20 degrees. Mediolateral compensating curve, should not exceed 10 degrees

Studies have been done to record the forces exerted by muscles of mastication while chewing. The results in denture patients are extremely significant as due to the loss of individual teeth there is also resultant proprioception loss. The complete denture prosthesis wearers exert a maximum of 10 to 15% force in comparison to the individuals with natural teeth.

Therefore, the shape of the artificial teeth along with the occlusal scheme play a vital role in enhancing some efficiency while eating. The clinician must choose the correct occlusal scheme taking all the factors such as ridge condition, ridge relation soft tissues and others into consideration giving the patient a stable, unrestrictive occlusion.

## Need of Balanced Occlusion: A Controversy

Earlier and even now there has been a great debate over the need of balanced occlusion in complete denture cases. Many studies have

## Step 6 Occlusion

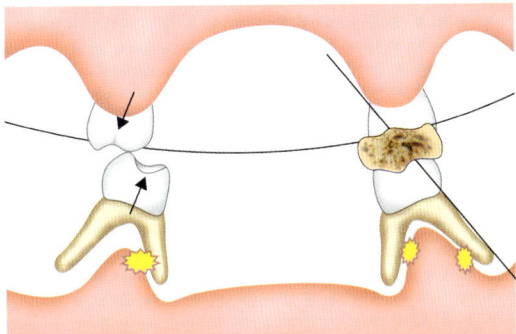

Fig. 6.14: Need of Balanced occlusion: Bolus in, Balance out

been done which prove that though in some patients balance does improve denture stability, the results are too small to be rendered significant. Balanced denture is still the preferred occlusal scheme and the norm since a long time but lingualized occlusion is also getting accepted now showing exceptional results **(Fig. 6.14)**.

## OCCLUSAL SCHEMES

### Bilateral Balanced Occlusion

- Aim:
  - Stable simultaneous multiple contacts of the maxillary and mandibular teeth in centric and eccentric movements which keep the denture stable **(Figs 6.15A and B, 6.16 to 6.19)**.
- Tooth Anatomy:

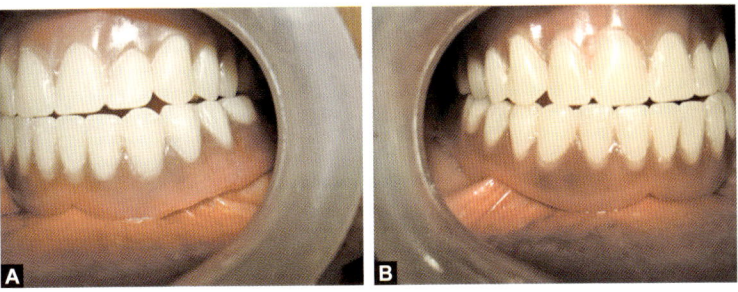

Figs 6.15A and B: (A) Bilateral balanced occlusion: Protrusive-contacts left side. (B) Bilateral balanced occlusion: Protrusive-contacts right side

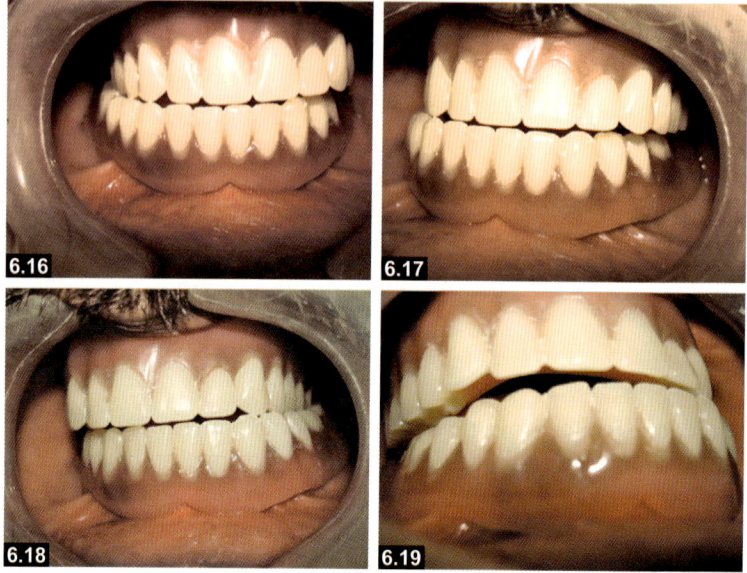

**Fig. 6.16:** Bilateral balanced occlusion: Right lateral working side. **Fig. 6.17:** Bilateral balanced occlusion: Balancing side. **Fig. 6.18:** Bilateral balanced occlusion: Left lateral working side. **Fig. 6.19:** Bilateral balanced occlusion: Balancing side

- Semi anatomic tooth mold preferred.

## Monoplane Occlusal Scheme

- Aim:
    - A ramp can be made posterior to the mandibular 2nd molar if balance is desired. Usually, no attempt is made to create balance in monoplane occlusion **(Fig. 6.20)**.

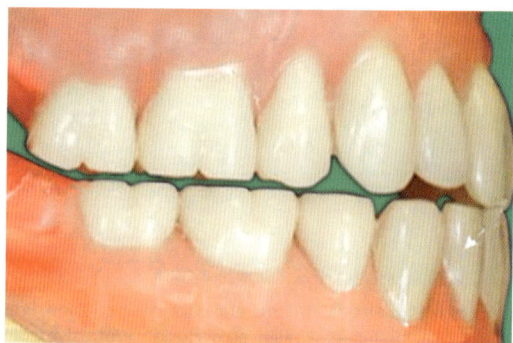

Fig. 6.20: Monoplane occlusal scheme (notice the ramp posterior to the 2nd molar to achieve balanced occlusion)

- This occlusal scheme is used to reduce lateral forces enhancing stability of the complete denture prosthesis
- Tooth Anatomy:
  - Non anatomic/zero degree cusp teeth.

## Lingualized Occlusion

- Aim:
  - Increased efficiency by maximizing upper palatal cusp contact with the lower fossa and marginal ridges. Reduced or buccally tilted maxillary buccal cusp with the widened mandibular fossa results in reduction of interferences and chances of denture instability **(Fig. 6.21)**.
- Tooth Anatomy:

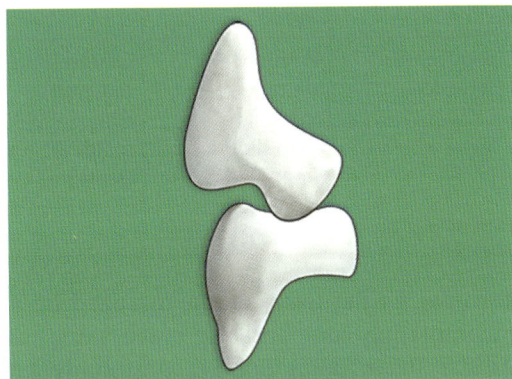

Fig. 6.21: Lingualized occlusion

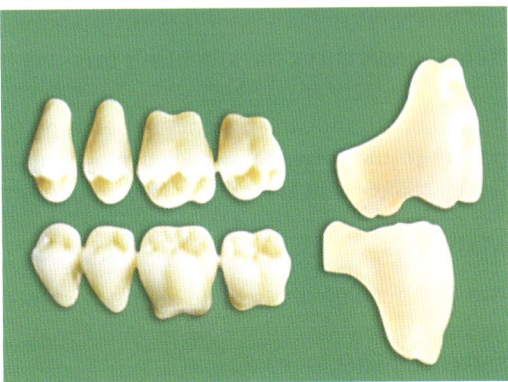

Fig. 6.22: Ortholingual denture teeth for lingual contact occlusion

○ Ortholingual molds designed specially for lingualized occlusal scheme. Smaller maxillary buccal cusp with wider and shallower mandibular central fossa **(Fig. 6.22)**.

## ■ OCCLUSAL CONCEPTS

| Concept | Advantages | Disadvantages | Tooth Mold |
|---|---|---|---|
| Bilateral Balanced Occlusion | Better chewing efficiency than other schemes. More natural appearing teeth | Time consuming with restriction of tooth positions due to locking of teeth | 20 degree cuspal angle |
| Monoplane Occlusion | Simplest with no lateral stresses. Easier for patients with neuromuscular deficit | Less esthetic with reduced efficiency in mastication | Zero degree teeth |
| Lingualized Occlusion | Reduced denture instability with slightly improved chewing efficiency | Customizing required if ortholingual molds are not available | Ortholingual mold |

Zero degree/flat teeth can be arranged in balanced occlusion by incorporating compensating curve along with a posterior ramp. Atleast three point contact posteriorly and anteriorly during protrusive movement is achieved.

**Note:** Always check the articulator from the back and visualize the cuspal contacts from the inside. Buccaly the contacts may look perfect but the actual efficiency depends on the contact of maxillary palatal to the lower fossa which may need correction before the teeth arrangement is ready for tryin appointment **(Fig. 6.23)**.

## Materials

Use of porcelain in complete denture prosthesis is almost obsolete as these materials cause a significant amount of bone loss/damage and are difficult to repair.

**Step 6** Occlusion

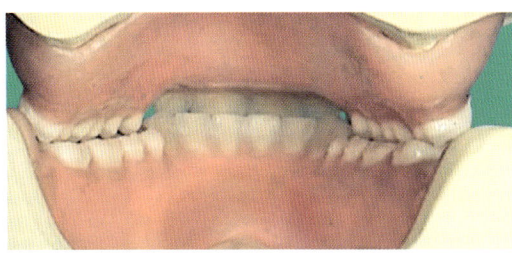

Fig. 6.23: Articulator from the back, visualizing the cuspal contacts from the inside

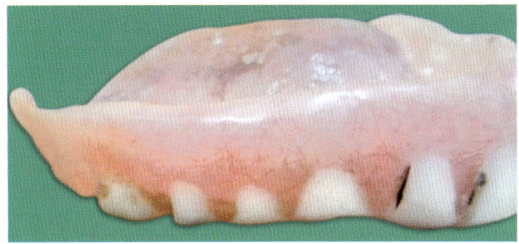

Fig. 6.24: Attrited acrylic denture teeth

Acrylic though widely and most commonly used gets attrited with time **(Fig. 6.24)**. Therefore, composites and metal onlays have been suggested for usage in cases showing bruxism and severe denture tooth wear.

Newer cross linked, high strength acrylics have been developed and their future as posterior teeth in complete dentures is promising.

## Conclusion

- Any occlusal scheme factoring in all the intra oral conditions can be used with satisfactory results ie: retention, support and stability.
- Balanced occlusion is still the preferred occlusal scheme, even though the differences between balanced and regular teeth arrangement are statistically not significant.
- Acrylic resin teeth are the most common posterior tooth material used. Reinforced acrylic teeth are stronger as they are more resistant to wear and have now replaced simple crosslinked basic acrylic teeth of the past.
- Porcelain teeth have been shown to cause severe bone loss of the residual ridges, thus are not used regularly in complete dentures.

# Step 7

## Laboratory Communication

*"The insertion appointment is the process of eliminating errors."*
F. J. Kratochvil

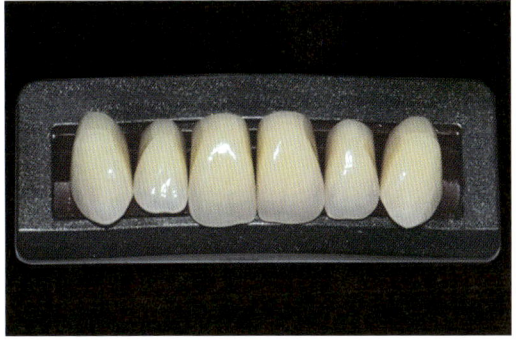

# Step 7

# Laboratory Communication

## INTRODUCTION

The success of any prosthesis depends not only on the high quality clinical work done by the dentist but also on the other unseen partner, i.e. the laboratory technician. The other factors involved are:
- The condition of the oral tissues and anatomy
- The material to be used
- Clinical skill of the dentist
- Patient expectations.

As the work has to be sent to the laboratory for fabrication of the prosthesis and intermediary steps, it is imperative that the dentist has a good working relationship with the laboratory technician.

Many a times verbal instructions may be necessary for better understanding but the written aspect is fundamental to proper communication, record keeping as well success of the final prosthesis. The work authorization letter can be either hand written, customized for a difficult case or a prewritten form.

Clinicians prefer a prewritten form in most of the complete denture cases due to the following reasons:
- Neat and clear
- Concise
- Standardization
- Saves extensive writing due to presence of checkboxes

- Time saving
- Complete
- Can be customized
- Ensures clinician does not forget anything important
- Easier for record keeping and maintenance
- Legal documentation.

A basic laboratory procedure work authorization form for any prosthetic work must contain the following information:
- The name and contact details (phone number and address) of the laboratory
- The name and contact details (phone number and address) of the dental clinic
- Patient name and details such as age and sex
- The date of work authorization
- Instruction section
- The desired date of work completion
- Dentist/authorized personnel signature
- Registered license number.

It is mandatory to prepare authorization forms in duplicate so as to send the original to the laboratory whereas a copy is to be maintained in the dental office. Effective communication (written + verbal), cooperative professional relation and mutual respect between the dentist and the laboratory technician are the corner stones to build a successful prosthesis. The importance of the same cannot be emphasized enough.

The written directions to the laboratory technician for each procedure if done through a detailed, meaningful work authorization form and verbal communication (if required) will ensure professional quality leading to dentist and patient satisfaction. A legible, simple, concise and clear work authorization form is the dentists responsibility and can not be neglected.

Henderson suggested a simple, specific and complete laboratory procedure authorization chart for complete denture cases **Table 7.1** and another simpler version for laboratory communication is depicted in **Table 7.2**.

## Step 7 Laboratory Communication

**Table 7.1:** Henderson's complete laboratory procedure authorization chart

### COMPLETE DENTURE PROSTHODONTICS LABORATORY PROCEDURE AUTHORIZATION

To:
- Name _____
- Address _____
- City _____ State _____ Zip _____

Patient _____ Date _____

**Laboratory Procedure**

| | |
|---|---|
| Custom trays _____ | Record bases _____ |
| Occlusion rim _____ | Anterior tooth arrangement _____ |
| Posterior tooth arrangement _____ | Wax-up for try in _____ |
| Wax-up -- processing _____ | clear surgical template _____ |
| Occlusal index _____ | Mount maxillary denture _____ |
| Finish for delivery (except borders) _____ | occlusal equilibration _____ |
| Remount cast _____ | Repair _____ |
| Mount mandibular denture _____ | Rebase _____ |
| Reline _____ | Other _____ |

Deliver _____
               day        time

**Special Instructions**

(use back side for further instructions)

From: Dr. _____

Address _____

City _____ State _____ Zip _____

License Number _____ Phone Number _____

                                                               Dentist's Signature

### TEETH

| | ANTERIOR | Manufacturer | Mold | Shade | Plastic | Porcelain | Arrangement |
|---|---|---|---|---|---|---|---|
| MAX | Central | | | | | | |
| | Lateral | | | | | | |
| | Cuspid | | | | | | |
| MAND | Central | | | | | | |
| | Lateral | | | | | | |
| | Cuspid | | | | | | |

| POSTERIOR | Manufacturer | Mold | Shade | Plastic | Porcelain | Arrangement |
|---|---|---|---|---|---|---|
| Maxillary | | | | | | |
| Mandibular | | | | | | |

Special Teeth _____

### MATERIALS

| Casts | plaster _____ | stone _____ | improved stone _____ | |
|---|---|---|---|---|
| Trays | plastic patty _____ | plastic sprinkle-on _____ | plastic vacuum formed _____ | |
| Record Base | plastic patty _____ | plastic sprinkle-on _____ | plastic vacuum formed _____ | shellac _____ |
| Denture Base | Manufacturer _____ | | shade _____ | |
| Curing Cycle | Cold cure _____ | pour _____ | heat cure/long cycle _____ | heat cure/short cycle _____ |

Table 7.2: Laboratory communication chart

| Complete Denture work authorisation chart | | |
|---|---|---|
| Laboratory Name:_____ <br> Contact Number:_____ | Address:_____ <br> _____ | Contact Person:___ <br> _____ |
| Name Dr: _____ <br> Contact No:_____ | Address: _____ <br> _____ | Contact Person:___ <br> _____ |
| Patient Name: _____ <br> Sex:_____ | Age: _____ | Sign:_____ |
| **Complete Dentures** | **Work authorisation Date** _____ | **Work completion Date** _____ |
| **Laboratory Procedure:** <br> Custom trays: <br> Occlusal rims: <br> Anterior Tooth arrangement: <br> (Mold/shade/size) <br> Posterior tooth arrangement: <br> Wax up for tryin: <br> Finished denture for delivery: <br> Remount cast/Occlusal equilibration: <br><br> **Repair:** <br> Midline fracture: <br> Single tooth fracture/ replacement/addition <br> Other_____ <br> _____ <br> **Reline:** | *Maxillary*   *Mandibular* | Characterisation: <br><br><br><br><br><br><br><br><br> Material instructions: <br> _____ <br> _____ <br> _____ |

# Conclusion

- Due to multiple procedures and patient visits, complete denture treatment requires good communication between the dentist and the technician.
- Every clinician should have a customized work authorization form to ensure best results.

# Step 8

## Denture Insertion

*"The insertion appointment is the process of eliminating errors."*
F. J. Kratochvil

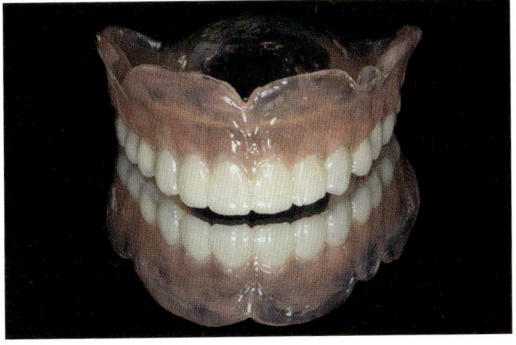

# Step 8

# Denture Insertion

## INTRODUCTION

The main objective of denture prosthesis in an edentulous patient is to rehabilitate the complete stomatognathic system including mastication, esthetics, phonetics. The dentures not only play a role in function but also help in uplifting the overall quality of our patient's life. Presence of well fitting and esthetically satisfactory dentures instills self esteem and confidence. A broader approach results in more patient centric dentistry **(Fig. 8.1)**.

## BEHAVIORAL FACTORS

As classified by Dr. Milus M. House, there is a vast spectrum of behavioral types in patients. Some are positive towards the

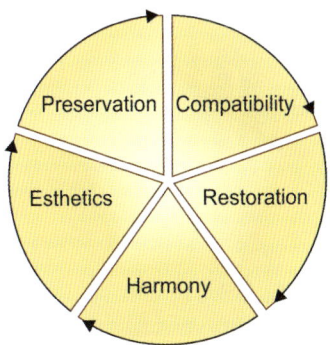

Fig. 8.1: Review of denture requirement

treatment and are easily satisfied where as a select few are just not in the mind frame to adapt to the new prosthesis.

## House Mental Classification for Edentulous Patients

Four groups depending on their psyche, past dental experiences and expectations:
1. Philosophical
2. Exacting
3. Hysterical
4. Indifferent.

Understanding patient's psychology during the first few sessions can help the dentist realize, patient's specific needs and prognosis of the treatment.

Ideally, the laboratory should return the dentures on duplicated, articulated and mounted casts **(Figs 8.2 to 8.4)**. The dentures should be first checked extra orally before even contemplating placing them in the oral cavity. Errors can be either technical from the laboratory/technician side or clinical ie: by the dentist. Assuming that the clinician has followed all the steps correctly, the processing errors need to be checked meticulously.

The bigger issues such as warpage, tooth movement due to compression molding, inadequately closed flasks and other such problems can result in substandard dentures.

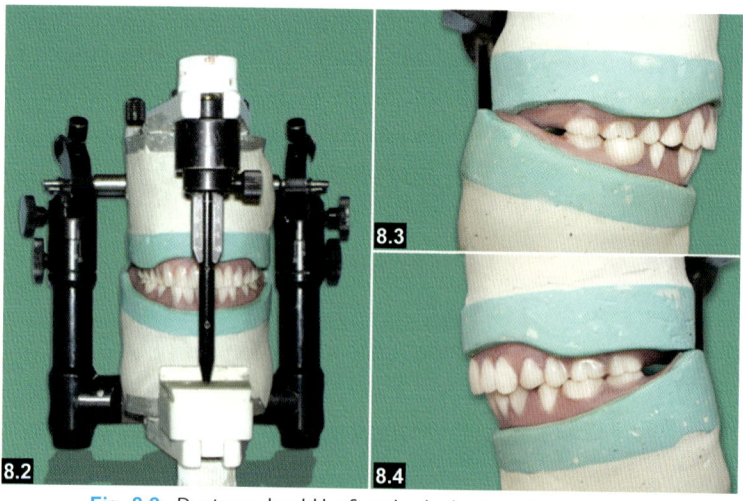

**Fig. 8.2:** Dentures should be first checked extraorally: front view.
**Fig. 8.3:** Right lateral view. **Fig. 8.4:** Left lateral view

**Step 8** Denture Insertion

## Suggested Extra Oral Checks
### Tissue side/intaglio
- Sharp, irregular, rough projections **(Fig. 8.5)**
- Bubbles/voids/nodules
- Presence of plaster/stone **(Fig. 8.6)**
- Scratch marks due to poor handling
- Unnecessary polishing of the tissue surface **(Fig. 8.7)**.

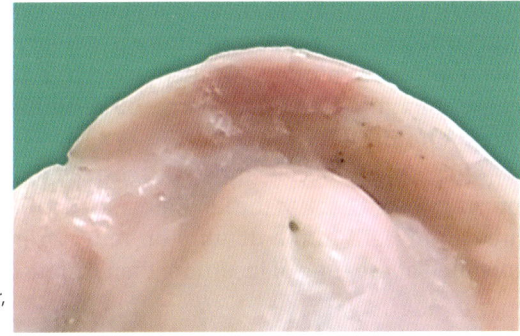

**Fig. 8.5:** Sharp, irregular, rough projections

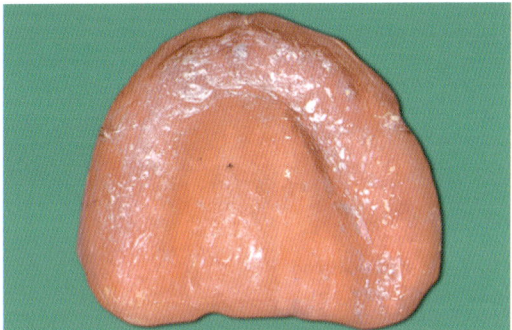

**Fig. 8.6:** Presence of plaster in the impression surface

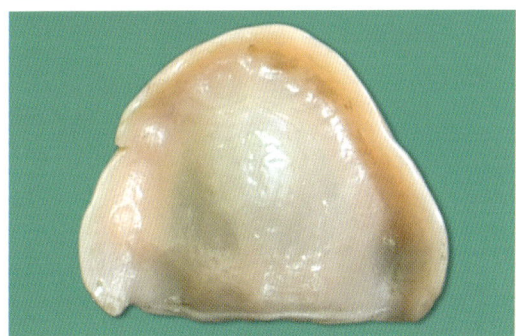

**Fig. 8.7:** Unnecessary polishing of the tissue surface

## Polished Surface/Cameo

- Poor polishing leading to unsightly scratch marks **(Fig. 8.8A)**
- Contouring of the surface
- Denture Periphery: Underpolished/Overpolished
- Presence of plaster in interdental areas **(Fig. 8.8B)**.

The above mentioned problems may lead to patient discomfort and compromised denture esthetics and function. Sharp edges and nodules cause immediate pain on insertion where as bubbles, scratches and voids create food lodgment. Under polished borders and surfaces may result in denture instability as the tissues do not adapt properly around the denture. Over polished borders can cause thinning of the peripheral roll resulting in reduced denture retention **(Fig. 8.9)**.

Such inadequacies must be corrected at the clinic or the prosthesis sent back to the laboratory for correction. If discrepancies are still present in the denture on return from the laboratory and tolerated at the time of insertion, then inspite of the efforts taken by

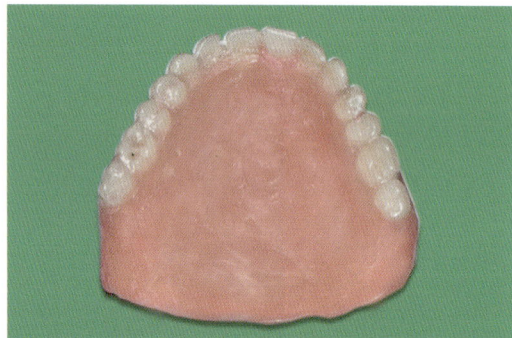

Fig. 8.8A: Poor polishing leading to unsightly scratch marks

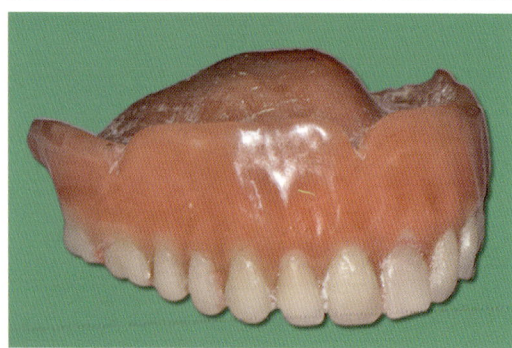

Fig. 8.8B: Presence of plaster in interdental areas

## Step 8 Denture Insertion

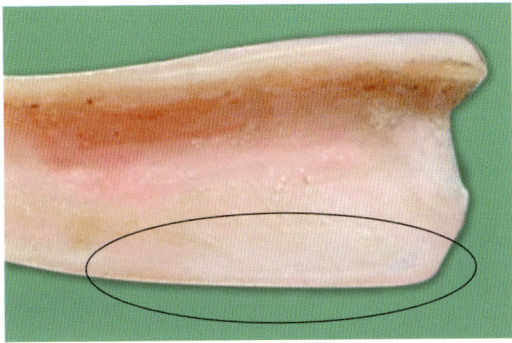

Fig. 8.9: Thinning of the peripheral roll due to over reduction and finishing by the laboratory/dentist

the clinician the patient will be unhappy and the prosthesis will be considered unsuccessful.

## Intra Oral Checks

Once the clinician is satisfied with the prosthesis and all the extra oral checks have been done, the dentures are inserted and evaluated individually.

Common maxillary and mandibular denture areas which may need adjustments are as follows **(Figs 8.10 and 8.11)**:

### *Maxillary Denture Areas*

- Frenum areas: Need to be relieved adequately : labial and buccal **(Fig. 8.12)**
- Disto-buccal flange: Presence of undercuts
- Acrylic beyond the posterior palatal seal area: Over extension is very common posteriorly
- Incisive papilla region: Insufficient relief **(Fig. 8.13)**.

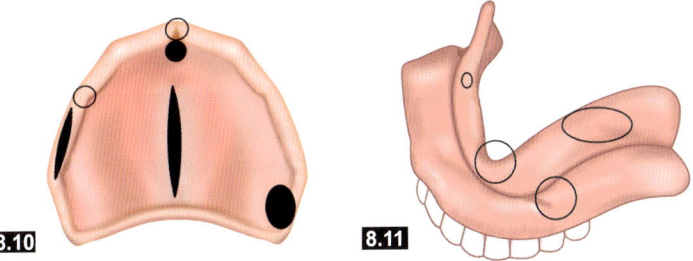

Fig. 8.10: Common maxillary denture areas which may need adjustments.
Fig. 8.11: Common mandibular denture areas which may need adjustments

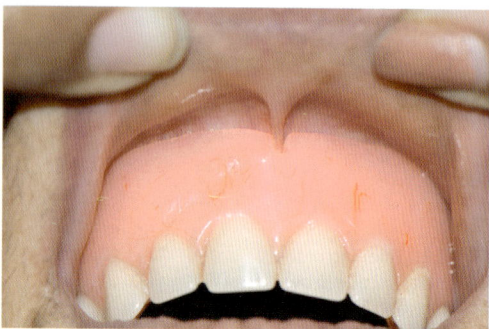

**Fig. 8.12:** Labial Frenum to be relieved adequately to avoid ulceration and pain on denture insertion

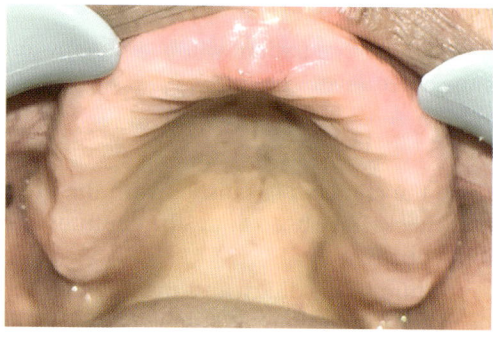

**Fig. 8.13:** Prominent incisve papilla. Naso palatine nerves and vessels pass through it. If not relieved adequately can cause pain, ulceration and parasthesia

## *Mandibular Denture Areas*

- Frenii, specially the lingual frenum: To be relieved
- Mylohyoid Ridges: Sharp ridges to be relieved or in presence of undercuts in prominent ridges
- Mental foramen: Prominent in resorbed ridges
- Genial tubercles: Need relief, if they become prominent in resorbed ridges.

## Various Intraoral Checks are as Follows

- Adaptation
- Border Extensions
- Relief areas
- Denture retention, stability and support
- Detecting the compressive areas
- Esthetic evaluation
- Verification of vertical and horizontal relation
- Occlusion
- Phonetics

## Step 8 Denture Insertion

### Adaptation to Tissues

- If the denture base does not adapt satisfactorily to the underlying mucosa, it can lead to loss of retention and unstable dentures. Dissatisfactory, definitive impressions or technical laboratory errors can result in poor adaptation. Most common laboratory error is due to warpage of the acrylic processed denture base (if maintained) which undergoes re-processing during the final heat curing
- Solution: Relining or rebasing to be done only if other parameters such as occlusion, phonetics, esthetics are satisfactory. Minor adaptation problems can be corrected with relining whereas major warpage requires rebasing procedure **(Fig. 8.14)**.

### Border Extensions

- Over extended Peripheries:
    - Signs: If the retentive dentures become lose as soon as the patient relaxes or tries to speak or eat.
    - Solution: Check for over extensions either visually or utilizing PIP ie: Pressure indicating paste. Reduce the over extended areas which in turn should make the dentures more retentive **(Fig. 8.15)**.
- Under extended Peripheries:
    - Signs: The dentures are un retentive showing zero signs of developing a peripheral seal or suction. The posterior extensions in maxilla and mandible ie: tuberosity region and the retromolar pad area are common areas where under extensions lie.

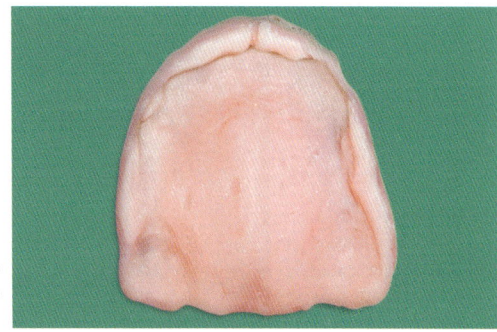

**Fig. 8.14:** Relined maxillary denture: Soft, chairside reliner used

- Solution: Any peripheral molding material such as green stick compound or silicon can be added at the under extended areas to check for improved retention. Once the areas are identified, they need to be border molded and sent back to the laboratory for relining.

## *Relief Areas*

- Areas where the nerves and vessels pass such as incisive papilla or the areas with sharp bony protuberances may result in pain or numbing effect on the mucosa causing discomfort to the patient if not relieved.
  - Solution: Check these areas with PIP and relieve these areas with a bur or mark them before sending to the laboratory where these areas can be adjusted **(Fig. 8.16)**.
    It is preferable to handle minor corrections in the clinic such as relieving 'localized' pressure points in the denture saving on time and added laboratory cost.

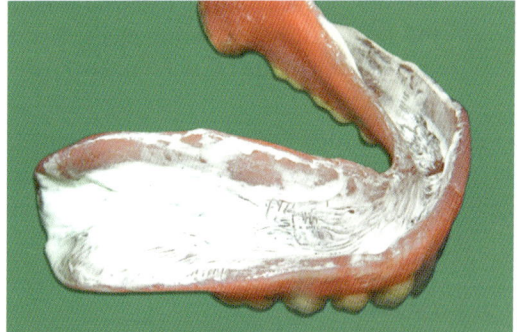

Fig. 8.15: Pressure indicating paste placed on a mandibular denture

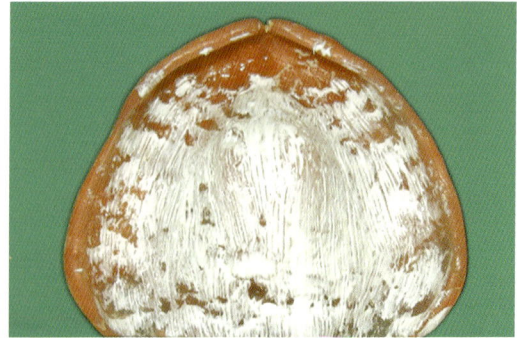

Fig. 8.16: Areas of compression indicated by Pressure indicating paste are relieved with a bur

## Denture Retention, Stability and Support

- Improper Posterior palatal seal (PPS) is one of the major reasons for loss of retention, stability and support. The PPS may be short, over extended or too thick/thin for the post seal to develop resulting in denture failure. Stability may get compromised drastically due to errors in occlusion as well, which will be discussed later.
    - Solution: Over extended and thick PPS needs to be reduced to the right space which would increase adaptation and enhance retention. If this does not work, check the PPS extension in the oral cavity by asking the patient to say "Ah" in short bursts. A space between the tissue and posterior extension means the denture may require development of the posterior seal again with the help of Green stick compound/silicon material. Once recorded, the denture must be sent back to the laboratory for acrylization of the added material.
    - Lack of time and inability to resend the work to the dental technician can be handled by using light cure/self cure acrylic in the PPS area. This will improve denture retention but the cold cure acrylic will deteriorate faster than its heat cure counterpart.

## Compressive Areas

- Thick flanges along with areas of excessive pressure/compression result in denture sore spots, ulceration and patient discomfort. Large pressure areas may even result in excessive and overt loss of the alveolar bone which in time may lead to sharp, uneven, thin alveolar ridges which are difficult to restore with conventional methods. Such cases may require grafting at a later stage where as extremely severe cases where geriatric patients are also suffering from debilitating medical conditions are almost impossible to treat making them what is called as a dental cripple.
    - Solution: Soft tissue ulceration can be marked on the denture with the help of dyes(used with a brush) applied on the sore spot and the mark transferred to the denture, which is later relieved.
    - Pressure Indicating Paste (PIP) or disclosing wax is applied to the denture borders and the denture base to indicate pressure points/areas which are eventually relieved with the help of acrylic burs (**Figs 8.17 and 8.18**).

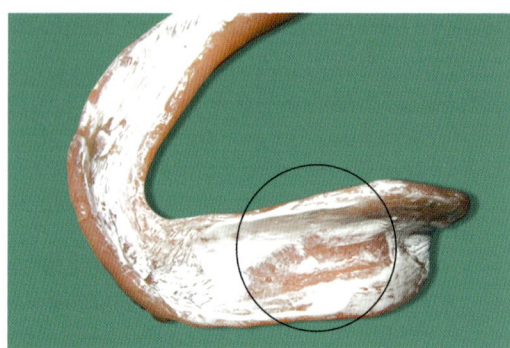

**Fig. 8.17:** Pressure points seen utilizing a pressure indicating paste in a mandibular denture

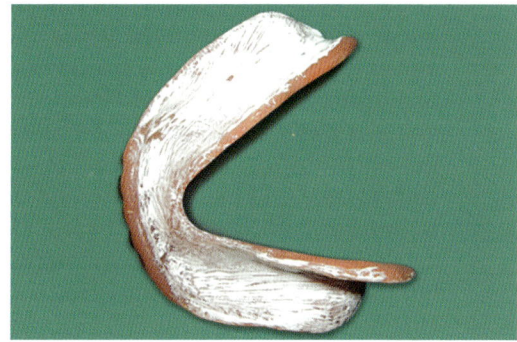

**Fig. 8.18:** Revealing no pressure points: Post correction

Once the pressure areas/points are removed, PIP is reapplied and the denture evaluated for areas where further relief may be required.

## *Esthetic Evaluation*

Natural shape, colour and placement of the denture teeth are reevaluated. Denture Characterization such as festooning, root carving, stippling done during try in stage is checked again intra orally along with the gingival colour characterization in the final prosthesis **(Fig. 8.19)**.

If the gingival shade is not as expected minor adjustments to the colour tone can be managed.
○ Solution: Dentures have to be sent back to the laboratory for adjustments where colour pigments are added and cured.

## *Errors in Vertical Dimension*

Both, excessive vertical dimension and over closure are problematic from a functional point of view.

## Step 8 Denture Insertion

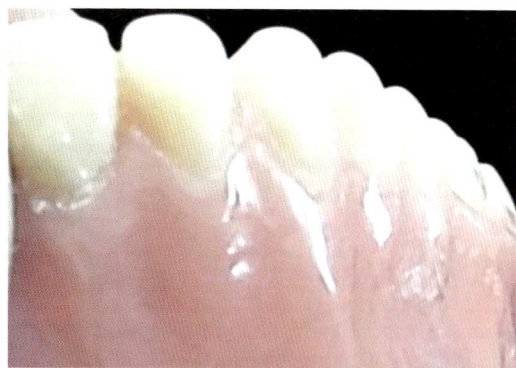

Fig. 8.19: Root carving

| Increased VD | |
|---|---|
| Speech gets compromised: Loss of freeway space and Silverman's closest speaking space<br>Clicking sound as teeth come in contact sooner than normal<br>Increased loss of residual alveolar bone<br>Trauma to the temporomandibular joint **(Fig. 8.20)** | 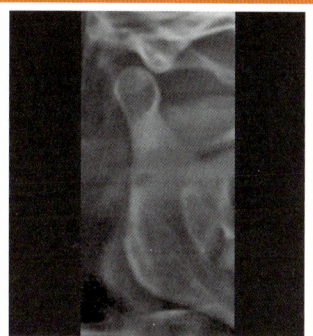<br>Fig. 8.20: Trauma due to icreased VD caused internal derangement |
| Inflammatory mucosa present all over the denture bearing tissues<br>Difficulty in swallowing<br>Inability to masticate comfortably<br>Long face syndrome: Compromised esthetics **(Fig. 8.21)** | 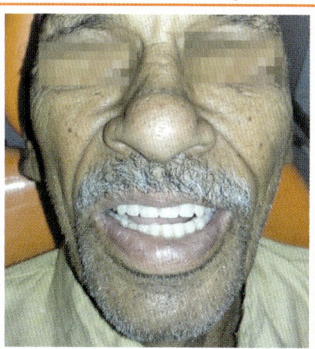<br>Fig. 8.21: Long face syndrome |
| Dry mouth: Lips parted at rest<br>Masticatory muscle fatigue | |

| Excessive Decrease in VD | |
|---|---|
| Inefficient masticatory capability due to reduced occlusal forces generated during chewing<br><br>Cheek biting and sometimes even tongue biting **(Fig. 8.22)** | 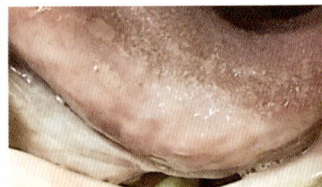<br>**Fig. 8.22:** Indentations of teeth on the lateral aspect of tongue |
| Prominent facial lines resulting in older appearance of the patient **(Fig. 8.23)** | 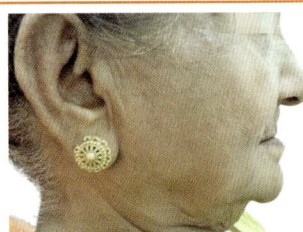<br>**Fig. 8.23:** Deeper facial lines resulting in older looking patient and a pseudo class III appearance |
| Smaller looking face<br><br>Drooping of the corners of the mouth causing dribbling of saliva **(Fig. 8.24)** | 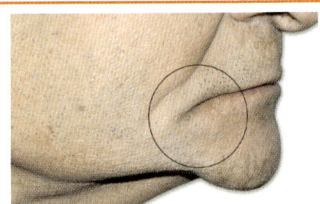<br>**Fig. 8.24:** Drooping of the corners of the mouth |
| Candidiasis<br>Angular chelitis **(Fig. 8.25)**<br>Pain in temporomandibular joint | 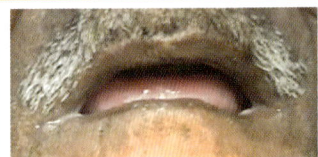<br>**Fig. 8.25:** Angular chelitis |

- Solution: Solution: Adjusting tooth surfaces to reduce the vertical dimension can only be done if the discrepancy is minimal. If such increase is excessive, then it is advisable to ask the laboratory technician to remove one set of the teeth and rearrange them. Anterior teeth can be utilized in remounting and resetting the posterior teeth to attain and maintain the vertical dimension.

## Step 8 Denture Insertion

The trial should be repeated and if the clinician is satisfied the denture is sent for curing.

### Errors in Centric Occlusion

- Once the denture base is fitting satisfactorily, denture occlusion is checked. The discrepancies such as premature or sliding contacts in occlusion if present will lead to loss of harmony within the stomatognathic system
- In theory, Bilateral balanced occlusion is the most accepted occlusal scheme for dentures ie: simultaneous three point contact of opposing arch teeth in the left and right posterior region along with anterior region during centric and eccentric movements. However, there is always a debate amongst clinicians on the necessity of balance in dentures
- Many of the early studies have given non confirmatory results about the need of balanced occlusion in complete dentures. Some authors even propagate canine guided occlusion in dentures suggesting that retention of lower denture along with general esthetics and chewing ability are improved with this type of disocclusion. Inspite of the differences, all agree that due to the presence of para functional movements in many of our patients, a balanced denture may be more stable.
- There are various problems that may happen after curing and are discussed below.
    - Solution: As most pre maturities are found in posterior teeth, clinicians must limit reductions to the following areas of the tooth (**Figs 8.26A to E**):
        - Cusp inclines
        - Central fossae
        - Marginal ridges.

### Common Errors in Centric Occlusion

| Occlusal Discrepancy | Clinical Adjustment Suggested |
|---|---|
| Opposing teeth pair: Too long- resulting in disocclusion of remaining teeth | Fossa of the involved teeth are deepened |
| Opposing cusp tips of teeth: Tip to tip-resulting in disocclusion of remaining teeth | 1. Grind on the inclines to move upper cusp buccally and lower cusp lingually<br>2. Broaden central fossa<br>3. Narrow lingual cusp of upper teeth and buccal cusp of lower teeth |

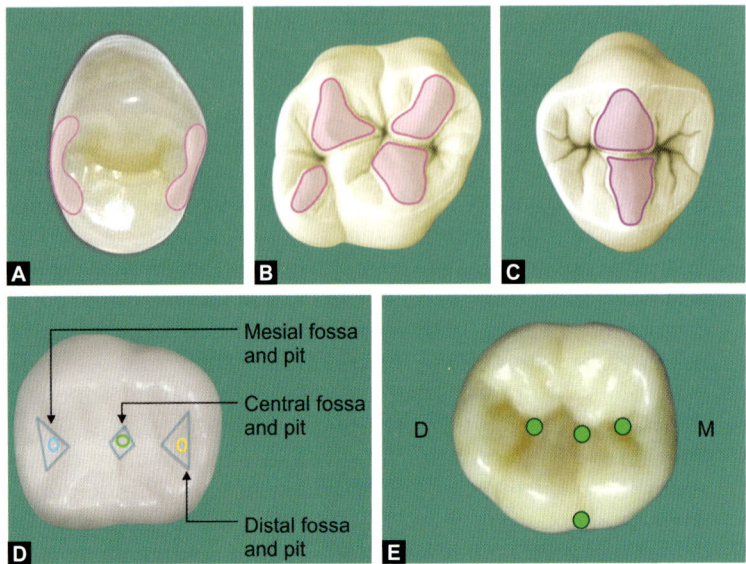

**Figs 8.26A to E:** Clinicians must limit reductions to these areas of the tooth

*Where to Grind First?*

The heaviest pre mature contacts always form a bulls eye with a dark ring surrounding a light center **(Fig. 8.27)**. These need to be eliminated first and the occlusion reassessed.

## *Phonetic/Speech Evaluation*

Excessive vertical dimension is a major cause for defective speech in denture patients. Other factors may be:
- Uneven or deficient palatal contour
- Incorrect arch form specially in the anterior region, constricted arch form
- Insufficient tongue space resulting in cramped tongue
- Poor retention/adaptation of final dentures, loose unstable dentures
- Teeth positioning: Silverman's closest speaking space.
    - Solution: All the above factors if in excess may need lot of changes/adjustments in the dentures with continual laboratory support and sometimes many steps need to be repeated to overcome the errors.

**Step 8** Denture Insertion

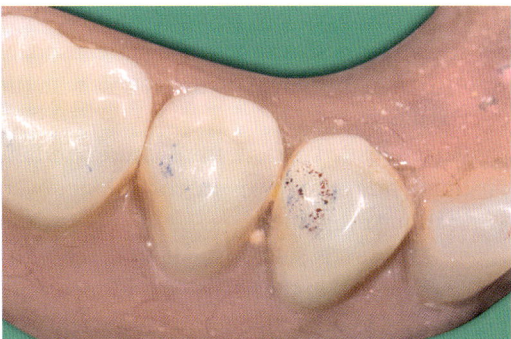

Fig. 8.27: The heaviest pre mature contacts always form a bulls eye

## Some More Dos and Checks

- Personalized palatal contour:
  - One aspect of customized characterization involves the duplication of rugae over the anterior part of the palate. This simulation helps those difficult patients adjust to the new dentures who are unable to do so and are more sensitive to changes in the oral cavity.
- Palatography:
  - It is a process of creating a customized palate for patients utilizing speech patterns. It is useful for patients who suffer from distorted speech patterns after a full mouth rehabilitation with complete denture prosthesis. Such patients who do not adapt to the new dentures even after a couple of weeks may require obtaining a palatogram and a customized complete denture accordingly
  - A palatogram is a graphic representation of the area of the palate contacted by tongue during a specified activity, usually speech-GPT 8
  - Any recording material can be used for palatography though use of a tissue conditioning material provides patient comfort, as well as sufficient working time for speech and tongue movement.

*Simple Method of Obtaining a Palatogram*

- Dry the palatal surface of the fabricated maxillary complete denture and place a tissue conditioning material on the palatal polished surface with the help of a brush

- Insert the maxillary denture and ask the patient to pronounce certain sounds ie the palatolingual consonants such as: s, sh, ch, n, k
- Also train the patient to use vowels with the consonents like cho, ko, sho
- Once satisfied remove the denture carefully without creating any finger prints on the tissue conditioner over the palate **(Fig 8.28)**.
- Marking evaluation:
    - Denture is sent to the laboratory with the new palatal form obtained in the tissue conditioner
    - Flasking is redone and an autopolymerising repair resin is used for customizing the palatal contours
    - Denture refinished and polished before delivery.
- Sibilant sounds and other consonants evaluated with the customized denture.

## Specific Speech Sounds

The common speech sounds are shown in **Figure 8.29**. The specific speech sounds and the words used to evaluate them are depicted in **Table 8.1**.

Table 8.1: Various speech sound and words for speech sound evaluation

| Speech Sounds | Words for Speech Sound Evaluation |
|---|---|
| S, sh | Sixty six, Mississippi, ship, sunshine, saraswati |
| T, D | Ted, Located, Noted |
| Ch, J | Church, join, challenge, Charles |
| K | Calcutta, duck |
| F, V | Five, fifty-five, vivacious |

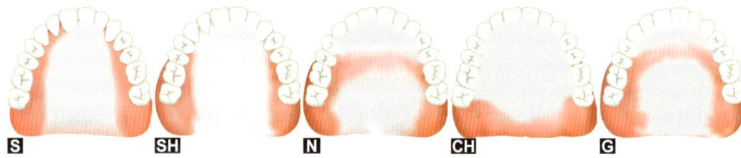

Fig. 8.28: Tongue positioning during various sounds, Palatogram

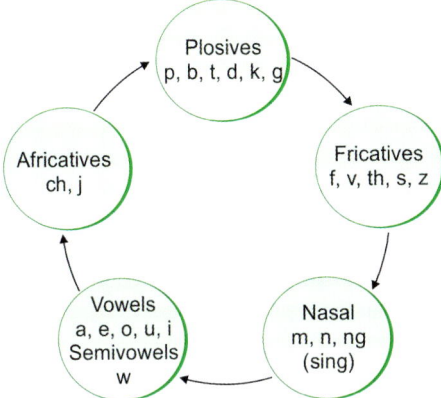

Fig. 8.29: Commonly used speech sounds, the consonants

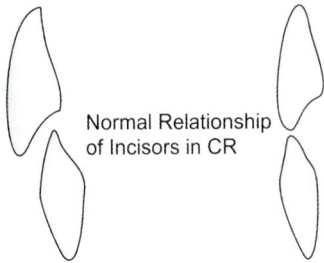

Fig. 8.30: Normal relationship of incisors in Centric relation and edge to edge (edges almost touching) relation when "S" sound is pronounced

## *Silverman's Closest Speaking Space*

Anterior teeth placement plays an important part in speech rehabilitation after complete denture delivery. Sibilant sounds such as "s and sh" are most affected.

When the patient pronounces "S" the maxillary and mandibular incisors must come edge to edge with out touching ie: minimal space is present which is known as Silverman's closest speaking space **(Fig. 8.30)**.

## Conclusion

- Denture insertion is not the end of treatment but just a final step where the prosthesis is given to the patient.
- Minor corrections are done chairside without changing the important parameters incorporated in the complete denture prosthesis. Dentures need to be reviewed within 24-48 hours of delivery to ensure patient comfort.
- Regular recalls for check ups, patient motivation and ensuring that the patient adapts to the new prosthesis with co responsibility and cotherapy is what makes the treatment a success.

# Step 9

## Denture Maintenance with Patient Education

*"Educating the mind, without educating the heart is no education at all"*

*Aristotle*

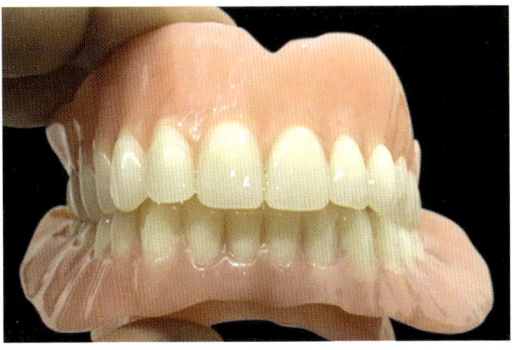

# Step 9

# Denture Maintenance with Patient Education

## ■ INTRODUCTION

Patient education starts from the first visit and continues till the final recall visits. After a thorough examination, patient should be made aware of the limitations of the treatment procedure. Many prosthetic treatments have failed in the past due to unrealistic patient expectations and miscommunication between the dentist and the patient.

Understanding patient expectations and discussing treatment outcomes with realistic results, helps in creating a positive patient attitude. Patient involvement during the treatment phase reduces post insertion problems due to communication gap and also makes the patient feel more responsible towards the treatment in a complete holistic way.

Communication at the time of denture delivery is critical. It is important to make the patient understand the problems he/she may face for a short while after denture insertion. Patients should be motivated to discuss their fears and encouraged to ask questions regarding the same.

Patient should be made aware of the following denture related facts before the final insertion appointment:
- Concept of mastication with new dentures
- Foreign feel
- Patient individuality
- Appearance with dentures in the oral cavity
- Excess salivary flow
- Speech with dentures

- Pains and aches with new dentures
- Tissue preservation
- Hygiene:
  - Denture hygiene
  - Oral hygiene
- Over the counter products:
  - Adhesives
  - Repair and Reline kits
  - Analgesic gels

## Concept of Mastication with New Dentures

Complete denture mastication is a slow, deliberate, methodical and programmed process which needs patience and practice. A chewing center is believed to be located with in the brain stem (reticular formation of pons) **(Fig. 9.1)**.

Many edentulous patients have a desire to test their new dentures immediately trying to check how well they function. It is the clinician's duty to advice patients about the chewing patterns, helping them develop their own chewing skills. Most of the times, new memory patterns for the muscles need to be made and adapted accordingly. Once they come into habit, patient is able to chew without any conscious effort.

Soft, non sticky food is preferred initially after insertion followed by crispy, easily chewable ones. Hard, fibrous foods are to be tried much later once the denture wearer has mastered the simpler foods.

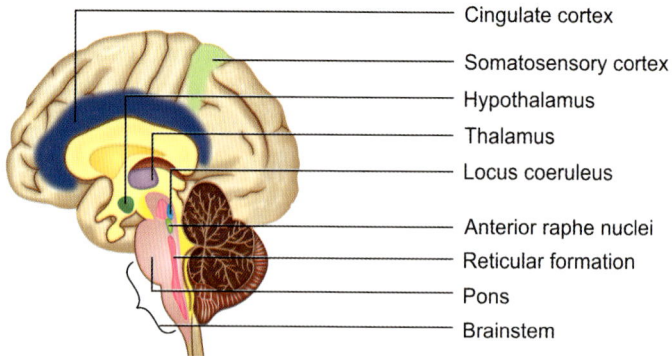

Fig. 9.1: Chewing center located with in the brain stem (reticular formation of pons)

Eating efficiency of patients with dentures though much lower than those with natural teeth is eventually a developed skill, which initially needs diet selection and motivation. Other factors which are not in the clinician's hands but effect mastication are:
- Patient age
- Residual ridge resorption stage
- Neuromuscular coordination
- Inter arch ridge relationship
- Tongue size and position.

## Foreign Feel

The first oral feeling after denture insertion is that of fullness or bulk. Ideally the patient should be explained that this foreign feeling with new dentures is normal and expected. Patient must be allowed to view himself/herself in the mirror as this instills a sense of confidence and reassures the patient.

Forewarned patients accept dentures better than those who have unrealistic expectations or those who have not been made aware of these new oral feelings. An educated and motivated patient is eager to accept the new dentures and face these small problems which will either fade away on their own due to familiarization or can be corrected by the dentist **(Fig. 9.2)**.

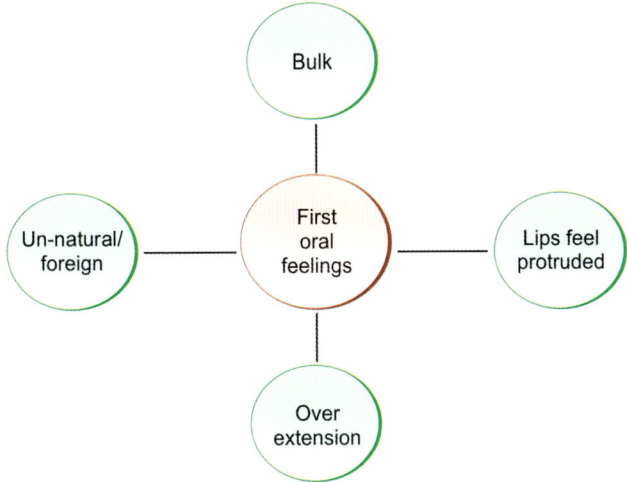

Fig. 9.2: Oral feelings with the new dentures

## Patient Individuality

Each patient is unique and this important fact must be driven home before denture insertion. If patients try to compare their complete dentures and their functions with fellow denture wearers there is bound to be dissatisfaction. Depending on various anatomical, physiological and individual factors each denture is bound to be different in look as well as function. Once the patient understands this and the limitations associated due to his specific conditions, the chances of denture acceptance are much higher.

## Changed Appearance with New Dentures

Patient's who have been edentulous for a long time show a remarkable change in appearance **(Fig. 9.3)**. Immediate denture patients or those with relatively short edentulous span are likely to maintain their facial appearance without much difficulty.

Older patients and new denture wearers sometimes find a drastic change in appearance due to stretching of circum oral musculature **(Fig. 9.4)**. It must be explained that with time the muscles will get adapted to and around the prosthesis resulting in a more natural looking face. The perceived bulk and excess will also improve and change with familiarity as tense muscles will relax and settle.

During long edentulous span, there is collapse of vertical dimension with unsupported lips and deepened facial line angles causing the patient to look older **(Fig. 9.5)**. Once the dentures are inserted, there is a marked positive change in patient appearance which is brought about by factors such as: restoring the vertical dimension, lip and cheek support, filling of the deepened lines and a pleasing smile **(Fig. 9.6)**. Patient's need to be informed of the changes so that they are mentally ready for the dentures and their improved appearance or else they may want to go back to their initial old look causing distress to the patient and the clinician.

## Excessive Salivary Flow

Salivary flow increases as soon as the dentures are placed in the oral cavity. The foreign feel of the dentures triggers the sensory neuro receptors causing stimulation of salivary glands. Patients must be made aware of the over active salivary flow and be educated about the need to avoid spitting and rinsing again and again as it causes

## Step 9  Denture Maintenance with Patient Education

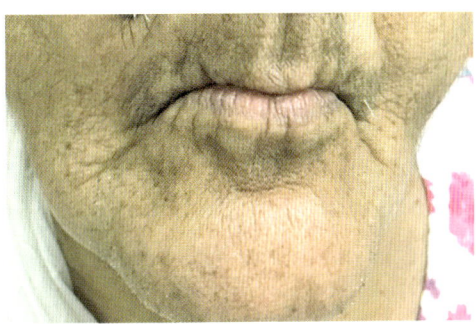

Fig. 9.3: Edentulous patient without dentures. Loss of circumoral support, exaggerated facial lines, wrinkles causing change in appearance are visible

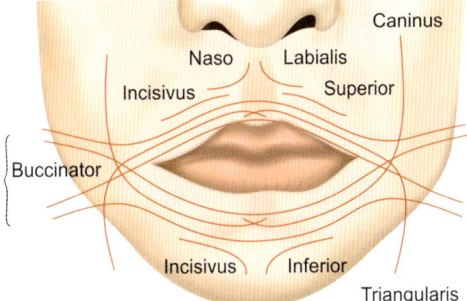

Fig. 9.4: Circumoral musculature

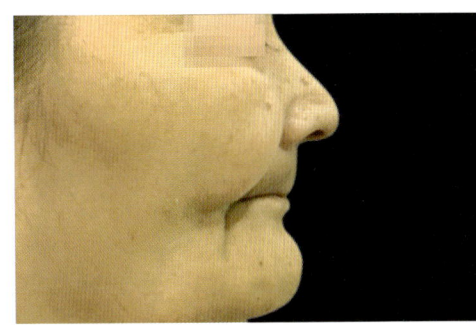

Fig. 9.5: Collapse of vertical dimension with unsupported lips and deepened facial line angles

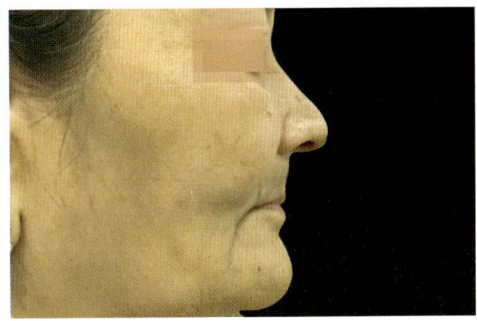

Fig. 9.6: Restored vertical dimension with complete dentures

denture instability. Swallowing the excess saliva is recommended. Once the body and the oral cavity gets familiar with the dentures ie: the dentures are no more new, the salivary flow reverts to normal. Ideally, 2-3 weeks is the time period told to patient in which the salivary flow normalizes but is variable.

## Speech with New Dentures

Owing to the odd first feeling of excess after denture insertion, speech discrepancy is normal and to be expected. Six valves are involved in speech and five of them affected by tooth position are as follows:
1. Bilabial (Not affected by tooth position)
2. Labiodental
3. Linguodental
4. Linguoalveolar
5. Linguopalatal
6. Linguovelar.

Distorted and unfamiliar sounding speech is usually an initial hindrance which should not act as a deterrent to patient motivation. An aware and educated patient will accept this challenge and practice till he sounds more like himself. It is recommended that the patient practices loud reading as it will help in fluency of speech and tone. Sibilant sounds are most commonly affected and are the last ones to be corrected.

It is advised to make patient speak full sentences in the clinic before allowing the patient to leave the clinic to instill confidence. Avoid being repetitive ie: making the patient say the same word which will make the patient conscious of the different sound making him/her uncomfortable and eventually demotivated.

## Pains and Aches with New Dentures

Soft tissue encasing the underlying bone is trapped between two hard surfaces and may react to pressure in the form of pain, ulceration or redness. Denture extensions in the vestibular sulci either push the muscles or get moved around resulting in abrasion and tissue irritation, causing pain.

It is advisable to remove the dentures out for some time if there is pain, to provide the much needed rest for healing. Sore spots can be identified and tackled by the clinician on recall appointments (**Figs 9.7 and 9.8**).

## Step 9 Denture Maintenance with Patient Education

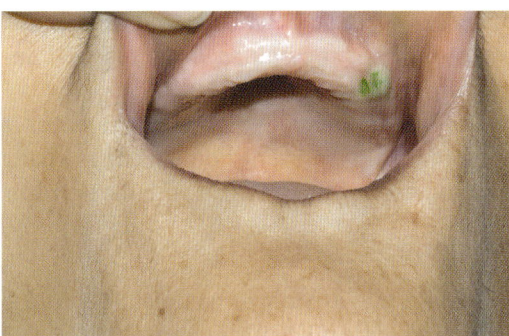

Fig. 9.7: Dye placed on the ulcer with a brush

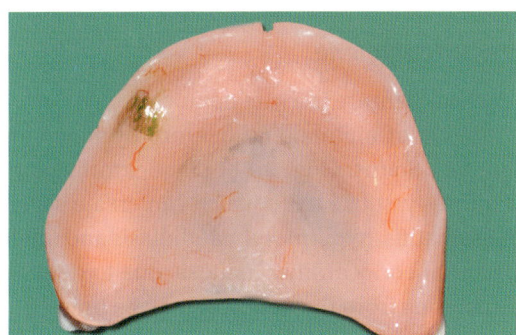

Fig. 9.8: Dye marking replicated on the denture for precise correction

Many a times the muscles of mastication and facial muscles get fatigued due to eating with new dentures. Some patients who have been edentulous for a long time, develop skills to chew food with tongue and alveolar ridges. These habits need to be unlearnt and such patients experience reduced chewing efficiency. With practice and time the new chewing pattern is formed and patients adjust to the dentures.

## Tissue Preservation

The patient is made aware, about the importance of tissue rest. Dentures need to be kept out of the oral cavity for atleast 6-7 hours per day as it allows the tissues to breathe. Failure to do so may result in one or all of the following:
- Severe bone resorption **(Fig. 9.9)**
- Epulis fissuratum: Inflammatory papillary hyperplasia due to constant irritation
- Candidiasis or other microbial/fungal infections
- Thin, friable mucosa
- Xerostomia: Dryness of mouth

It is observed that patients who wear dentures at night also show signs of bruxism resulting in increased bone loss and enhanced denture tooth wear **(Fig. 9.10)**.

It is recommended to place the dentures in a water filled closed container. This prevents dimensional changes which affect the denture making it last longer with the correct fit.

## Hygiene

There are two aspects to complete denture hygiene protocol and both have to be diligently followed.

### Denture Hygiene

"A clean denture is a safe denture".

Value of maintaining denture hygiene can not be emphasized enough. Stains, **(Fig. 9.11)** plaque, tartar and calculus deposit on dentures just like teeth which can create several health issues such as stomatitis, hyperplasia, candidiasis and other infections including bacterial endocarditis. Halitosis due to dentures and also bad odor emanating from the dentures may be present.

*Recommendations*

- Wash/clean dentures after every meal whenever possible with water and a soft denture brush on all surfaces
- Soaking in water mixed with a denture cleanser for a minimum of 30 mts/day to cause effective bacterial elimination. Full night soak is recommended
- Soaking in water without mechanical removal of debris will make the protocol ineffective
- Usage of tooth pastes for denture cleaning is to be discouraged as it can result in denture abrasion leading to scratches.

### Oral Hygiene

"The residual ridges were not created by God, to bear masticatory loads through dentures."

*Recommendations*

- Rinse the oral cavity thoroughly with water after every meal
- Cleaning the tongue with a soft brush every day

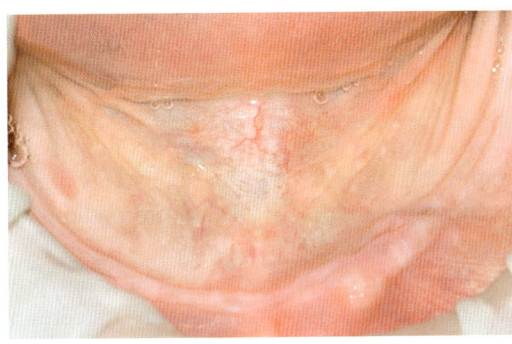

Fig. 9.9: Severe uneven ridge resorption

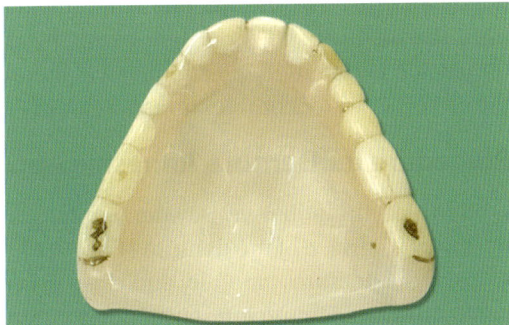

Fig. 9.10: Occlusal Wear caused due to night time denture wear

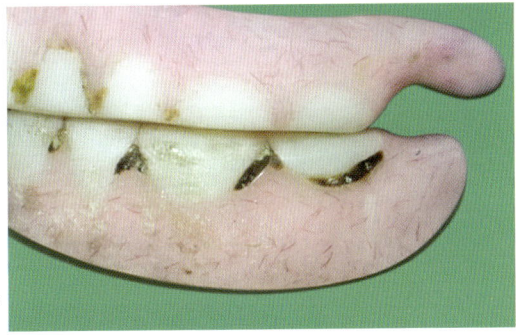

Fig. 9.11: Stains on dentures

- Massage the gingiva and the remaining denture bearing areas with the pad of the index finger twice daily (morning and night) to increase blood flow
- Non alcoholic Mouthwash is recommended.

## Over the Counter Products

Over the years, many self help complete denture products have come into the market.

## Adhesives

Use of adhesive powder or paste system to make an ill fitting denture retain is very common. Indian and American dental associations have accepted the use of many dental adhesives over the years. An important study by Woelfel et al states that "all denture adhesives occupy space". Thus, all denture patients are not good cases for adhesive usage.

Therefore, the adhesive must be given/prescribed by the dentist to enhance retention temporarily in certain cases but definitely not as a norm. Patients should avoid buying and using adhesives from the medical shops on their own. The discrepancy in vertical dimension and denture positioning will increase as the thickness of the adhesive-water combination increases **(Fig. 9.12)**.

## Procedure for Denture Adhesive Application

- Sprinkle the adhesive powder/apply paste evenly on the wet intaglio surface of the denture **(Fig. 9.13)**
- Seat the dentures carefully and close in centric relation position tightly at maximum intercuspation for thinning out the adhesive

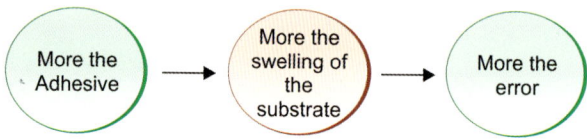

Fig. 9.12: Adhesive-error relationship

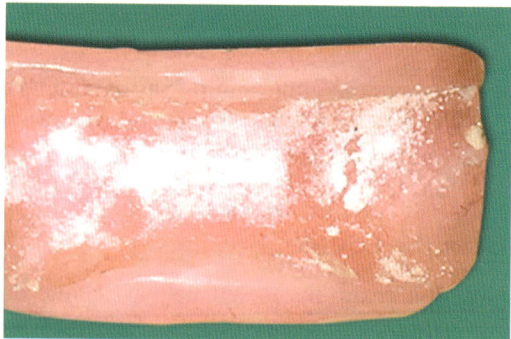

Fig. 9.13: Adhesive powder on the intaglio surface

### Step 9 Denture Maintenance with Patient Education

- After 30-60 seconds the patient can unclench as the denture is secure
- If adhesive needs to be re-applied, it is mandatory to wash out or brush out all the older adhesive particles before applying the next lot for better retention.

## Repair Kits

Self adjustment kits are the next common thing available and used over the counter by the patients. Two basic types:
1. Fractured tooth repair kit **(Fig. 9.14)**
2. Fractured denture base repair kit.

Unlike adhesives, repair kits are vehemently opposed by the dentists as many a times they mask the ill fitting denture symptoms and cause more harm to the underlying tissues.

Many patients still use such kits and attempt to repair their own dentures **(Fig. 9.15)** resulting in disastrous situations such as misaligned dentures and occlusal discrepancy.

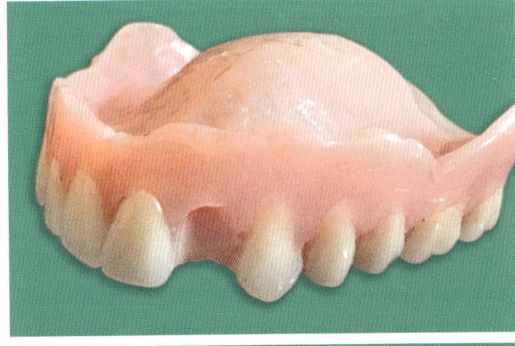

**Fig. 9.14:** Fractured dislodged tooth. Repair kits though available in the market are not recommended

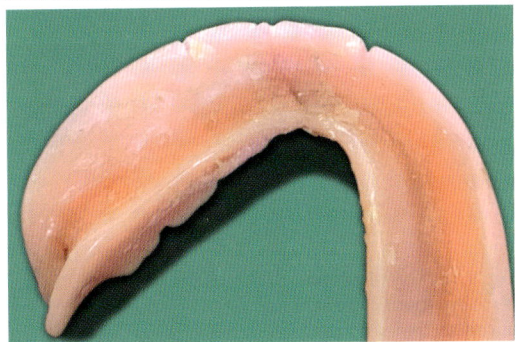

**Fig. 9.15:** Self repaired denture: Using an over the counter denture repair kit

## Reline Kits

Soft over the counter reliners cause vertical discrepancy, positional defects, retained odor and discolation of the dentures causing problems. It is advised to visit the dentist if the dentures becomes lose or don't fit rather than using such un reliable products **(Fig. 9.16)**.

## Analgesic Ointments

Ointments recommended by dentists maybe used to help reduce pain and heal. But applying such products to reduce denture soreness should only be used temporarily and not as a long term solution.

## Post Insertion Instructions in a Nutshell

Assurance that minor problems in new dentures are expected and can be detected early after a short interval of denture wear, alleviate patient apprehension. It also gives patient time to adjust to the new dentures. It is advisable to give written instructions to the patients to ensure compliance.

### *Post Insertion Instructions*

- Chewing:
    - Avoid rough, fibrous, tough foods initially. Start with soft, non sticky foods and slowly progress to harder ones
    - Eat slowly, methodoically and bilaterally as eating with complete dentures is a learned function
    - Do not try to bite food from the front teeth as it will lead to tipping/lifting of the dentures
    - Cut food into smaller pieces and place them directly on the posterior teeth for chewing.

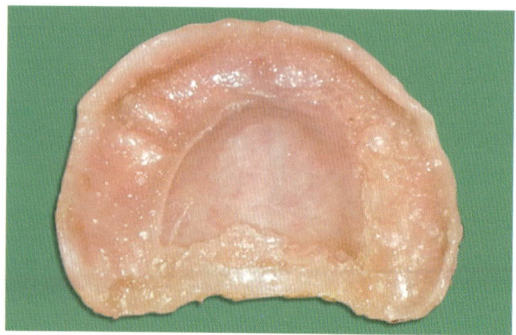

Fig. 9.16: Over the counter reline, causing change in vertical dimension and positional defect

## Step 9 Denture Maintenance with Patient Education

- Discomfort and pain:
  - In the event of denture pain, take the prosthesis out and rest the tissues
  - Wear the dentures again before the recall visit to make the sore spot detection easier
  - Do not panic as this can happen during the early stages of denture adjustments and will be tackled at the initial recall appointments.
- Excess salivary flow:
  - Increased saliva after wearing new dentures is normal and to be expected
  - This is triggered by the foreign feel of the denture which will normalize once the body gets familiar to the new prosthesis
  - Two-three weeks is the time period in which excess salivary flow will reduce but is variable in patients.
- Tongue coordination:
  - Avoid pushing the dentures out with the tongue as it should be used in stabilizing the lower denture, not making the denture un retentive
  - Ideally, the tongue should be in intimate contact with the lingual aspect of the mandibular denture keeping the denture in place
- Appearance:
  - Fullness and a change in appearance is to be expected in long span edentulous patients
  - With time the muscles will drape around the dentures and relax leading to a more natural appearance
  - Restoring the vertical may give a younger looking face.
- Speech:
  - Speech discrepancy initially is to be accepted and worked upon
  - Speak/read slowly and loudly in the comfort of home to improve fluency
  - Distortion of sibilant sounds usually takes longer to correct.
- Tissue Rest:
  - Dentures have to be removed from the oral cavity for atleast 6-7 hours/day
  - Do not wear dentures while sleeping
  - Massage the denture bearing tissues with the pad of the index finger daily.

- Foreign feel: The feeling of fullness and bulk will eventually settle once the oral cavity gets used to the new complete dentures with time.
- Denture maintenance:
  - Clean the dentures after every meal with water and a soft denture brush using non-abrasive pastes/cleansers
  - Dentures should be soaked in water mixed with denture cleansers at night
  - Avoid placing them in warm water as it tends to either bleach or distort the denture.
- Over the counter products: Avoid using over the counter products such as adhesives, relines or repair kits and analgesic ointments as they can lead to problems.

## Patient Recall

A well designed and fabricated complete denture prosthesis should require minimal adjustments during the initial recall visits. Patient's should be told that as the oral environment changes, the denture bearing tissues are subject to change. It is advised to have 12 month recalls for all denture wearing patients.

## Common 24 Hours Recall Check

| Problems | Problem Solving | Clinical Picture |
|---|---|---|
| Ulcers: Over extensions, sharp, overextended PPS bead **(Figs 9.17A and B)** Unrelieved frenii, sharp thin Mylohyoid ridge, | A dye can be used to mark the areas on the dentures. Apply the die with a brush on the sore spots and place the denture in the oral cavity. The dye markings get transferred which can be relieved in the dentures. | 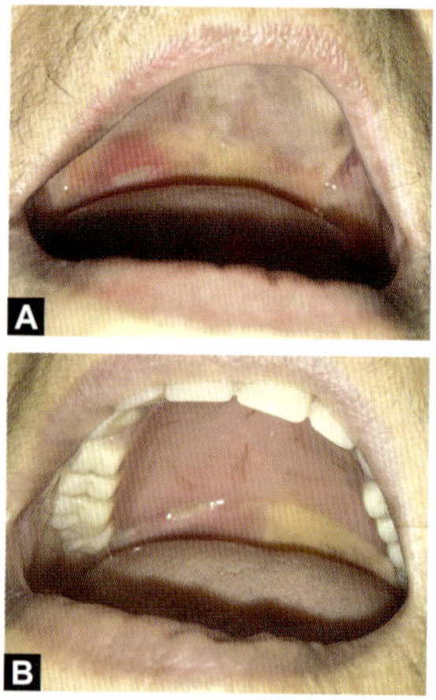 |

Figs 9.17A and B: (A) Ulcer due to over extended PPS. (B) Sharp, over extended PPS bead

## Step 9 Denture Maintenance with Patient Education 175

| | | |
|---|---|---|
| Soreness related to occlusion: pain on the slopes of the ridges due to deflective contacts | Occlusal equilibration is required **(Fig. 9.18)** | 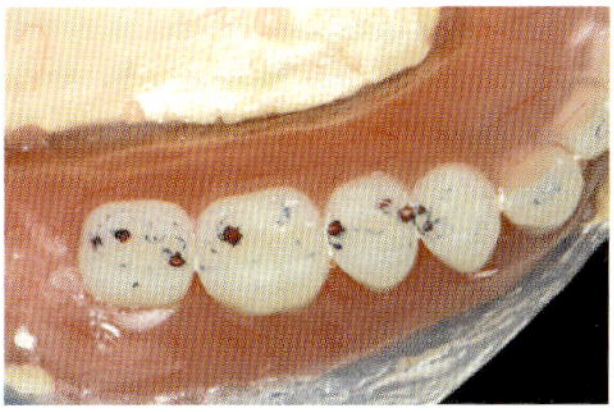 Fig. 9.18: Occlusal equilibration |
| Lose dentures: When the mouth is opened wide<br><br>Maxillary denture:<br><br><br><br><br><br>Mandibular dentures: | Check and relieve<br><br>- Distobuccal notch in the maxillary denture for coronoid.<br><br>- Distobuccal area in the mandibular denture for masseteric notch **(Fig. 9.19** | 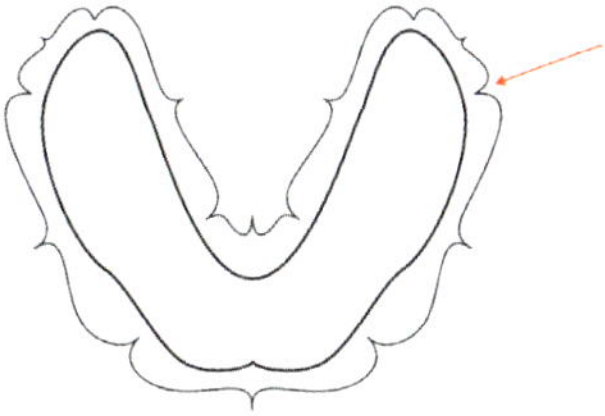 Fig. 9.19: Massetric notch |
| Over extended denture bases / excessive pressure areas | Pressure Indicating Paste (PIP): PIP: Pressure indicating paste is used. The areas of over extension or high pressure are relieved with a bur, the paste is reapplied and the checked for an even application of the PIP to ensure relief. **(Fig. 9.20)** | 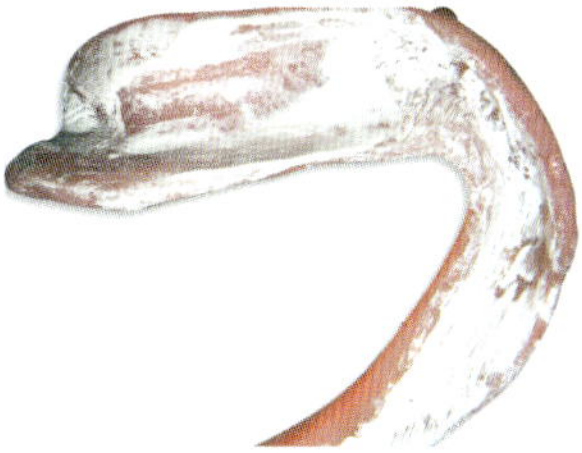 Fig. 9.20: Pressure indicating paste |

## Conclusion

- Understanding patient expectations and discussing treatment outcomes with realistic results helps patient adjust to the strangeness of new dentures.
- Clear instructions about denture maintenance need to be given to ensure clean dentures and healthy denture bearing tissues, to avoid denture related infections such as candidiasis.
- Communicating with the patient at the time of denture delivery will ensure that the patient does not panic when he/she suffers from any minor discomfort during initial adjustments.

# Step 10

## Special Techniques and Procedures

| | | |
|---|---|---|
| 10.1 | Immediate Dentures | 181 |
| 10.2 | Relining Procedures | 199 |
| 10.3 | Denture Repairs | 211 |
| 10.4 | Copy Dentures | 221 |

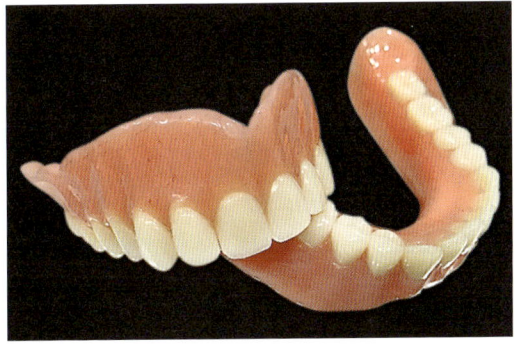

# Step 10.1

## Immediate Dentures

*"Every life deserves a certain amount of dignity,
no matter how poor or damaged the shell that carries it"*
                                           *Rick Bragg*

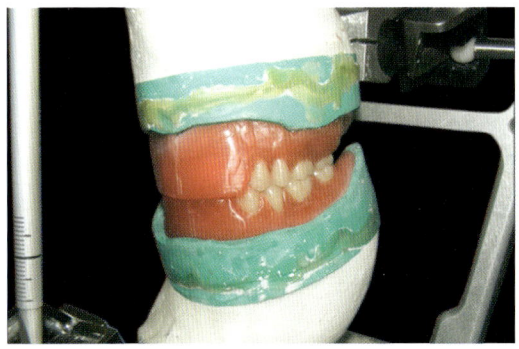

# Step 10.1

# Immediate Dentures

## INTRODUCTION

Replacement of teeth and surrounding associated structures as soon as they are lost. Though this procedure is not the norm, it is still done in many cases due to the various advantages especially from the patient's perspective.

Older patients many a times suffer from advanced periodontal disease, requiring multiple extractions. Such patients may not be comfortable with the edentulous state as apart from the loss of function, there is alteration in the patient's facial features making them unappealing in their own eyes. This is where any immediate prosthesis comes into play.

## DIAGNOSIS AND TREATMENT PLANNING

Once the patient's medical history is reviewed, a clinical, diagnostic and radiographic examination is done. It will reveal important factors such as:
- Periodontal condition of the remaining teeth and the extent of bone loss **(Fig. 10.1.1)**
- Presence of any retained root pieces, impacted teeth, foreign bodies
- Tori/exostoses/bony or soft tissue undercuts that need to be dealt with during the surgical extraction phase **(Fig. 10.1.2)**
- Positioning of the remaining teeth will help in determining discrepancies in the jaw relations and occlusal plane.

It is also important to understand patient's expectations, fears and overall psychological mind frame before fabrication of immediate dentures.

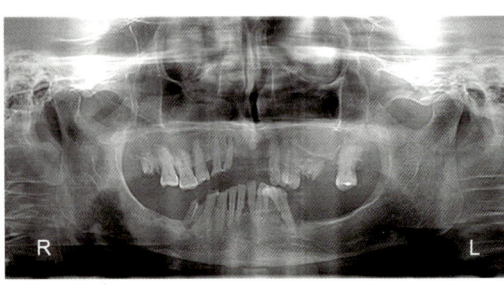

Fig. 10.1.1: Orthopantomogram of a peridontally compromised patient

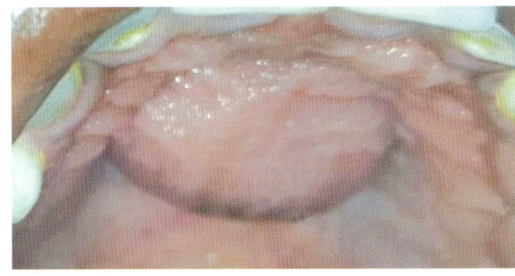

Fig. 10.1.2: Torus palatinus: Benign bony outgrowth in the palate

## TREATMENT STEPS

### Initial Impressions

Impressions can be made with alginate or silicon whichever material the clinician is comfortable with. In most cases, due to the presence of lose, supra erupted (periodontally compromised) teeth, there is a significant discrepancy between the teeth and edentulous areas causing the trays to rock. It is difficult to record adequate primary impressions with stock trays.

Trays need to be modified with wax or compound to ensure complete recording of both hard and soft tissues. Once an acceptable primary cast is obtained **(Figs 10.1.3A and B)**, a certain amount of space is given with the help of a spacer wax between the custom tray and the natural teeth. (2-4 mm usually).

### Final Impressions

The presence of remaining natural teeth makes this procedure a bit different than usual. Two techniques, i.e., Single tray technique and double tray technique have been most commonly used. These techniques have their merits and can be utilized in the situations where indicated. The clinician should be aware of them and be able to discern the situations where they can be used.

## Step 10.1 Immediate Dentures

### Techniques

- Single Tray Technique:
  - A single impression tray captures the natural remaining dentition along with the soft tissues simultaneously **Figure 10.1.4**
  - Impression formed with the help of this technique is shown in **Figure 10.1.5**.

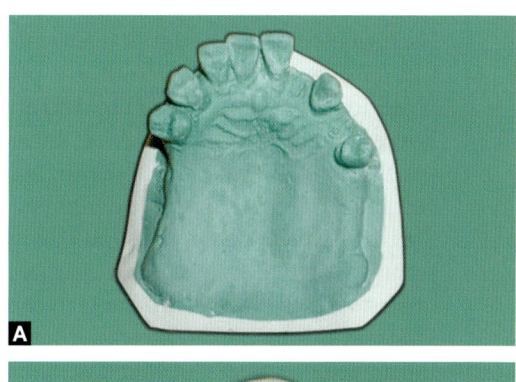
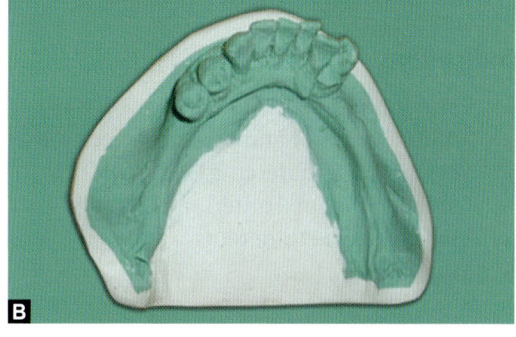

**Figs 10.1.3A and B:** Maxillary and mandibular primary casts: Clinically, remaining teeth showed grade three mobility. Wax sleeves were placed around the periodontally compromised teeth before making the primary impressions to ensure that the material loaded on the stock tray didn't lock around the teeth. This method ensures easy removal of the impressions without causing undue discomfort to the patient

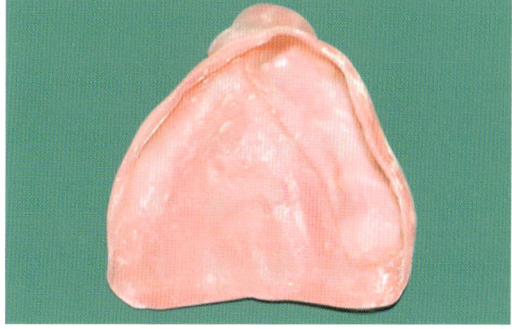

**Fig. 10.1.4:** Single tray technique: Single custom tray is used to capture both the soft tissues and teeth simultaneously

- **Double Tray Technique:**
  - The first tray captures the edentulous posterior soft tissues after which a second tray is placed over the first. This impression is called a pick up impression **(Figs 10.1.6 to 10.1.8)**
  - Better suited when the teeth are not compressible to maintain their positions during impression making
  - May also be utilized in severe periodontal cases where the teeth are mobile
  - Used when either anterior or posterior teeth are present
  - Can be used if anterior teeth are present with a bilateral posterior edentulous span **(Fig. 10.1.9)**
  - Border molding is done along the edentulous areas and the flange is extended over the dentulous area towards the vestibule to record complete peripheral extensions
  - First tray which covers only the edentulous zone is used to record peripheral extensions. A partial final impression (ZOE or elastomers) is made with the 1st tray after border molding.
  - First tray is then picked up with a 2nd tray that would record the anterior teeth at rest (Alginate or elastomers).

## Indications

- Periodontally stable teeth **(Fig. 10.1.10)**
- Multiple anterior and posterior teeth present **(Fig. 10.1.11)**
- Severe Labial undercuts **(Fig. 10.1.12)**
- Labially proclined anterior teeth **(Fig. 10.1.13)**
- Minimal tissue undercuts
- Mobile teeth.

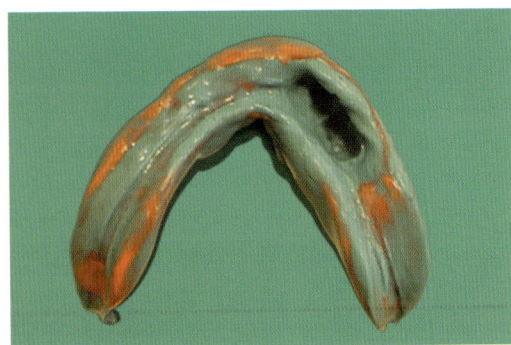

Fig. 10.1.5: Single tray impression, using elastomeric impression materials

## Step 10.1 Immediate Dentures

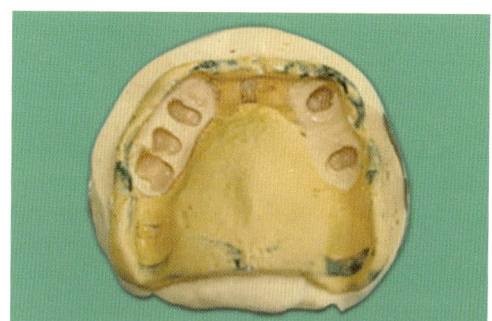

Fig. 10.1.6: Double tray technique: Two tray system used to record the maxillary arch

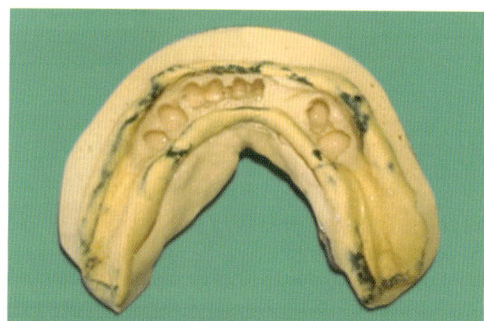

Fig. 10.1.7: Double tray technique to record the mandibular arch

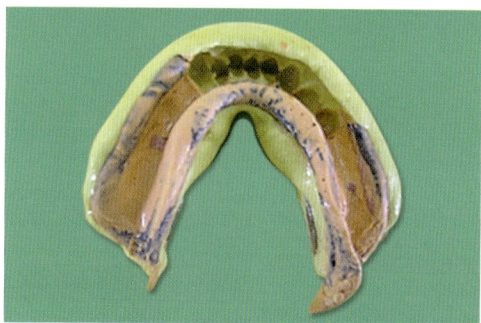

Fig. 10.1.8: Two stage impression: The 1st tray records soft tissues and the 2nd tray is used to record teeth. This impression also acts as a "pick up" impression

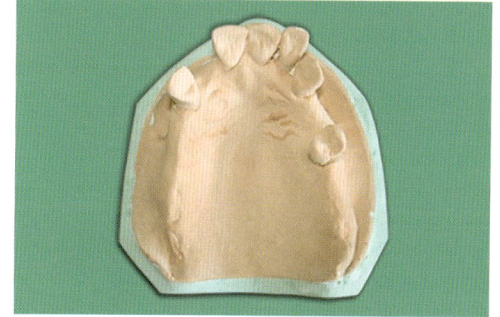

Fig. 10.1.9: Bilateral posterior edentulous span: Kennedy's Class I, modification 2

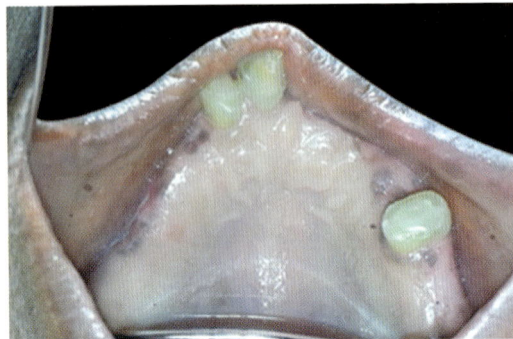

**Fig. 10.1.10:** Maxillary arch showing Periodontally stable root canal treated teeth with good bone support

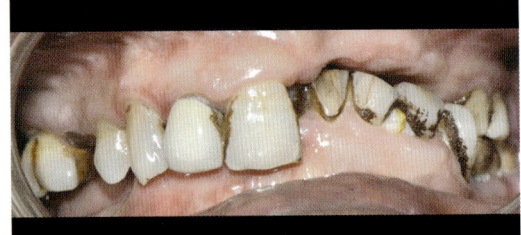

**Fig. 10.1.11:** Presence of multiple anterior and posterior teeth. Requiring 2 stage extractions. Posterior teeth are extracted first (pre denture fabrication extractions)

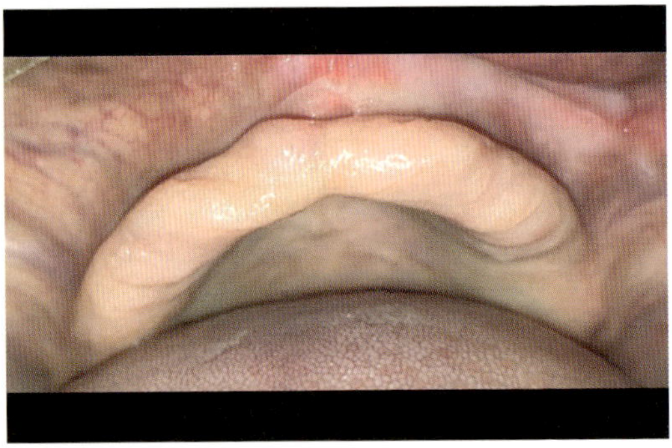

**Fig. 10.1.12:** Labial undercut: Bony prominence of the maxillary anterior ridge

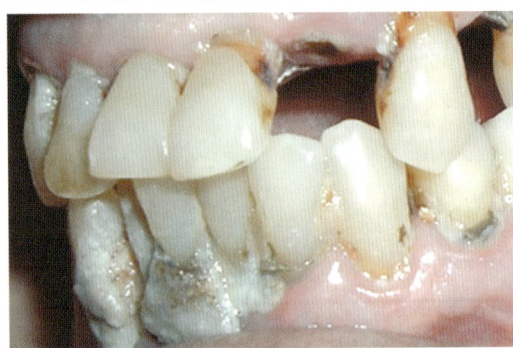

**Fig. 10.1.13:** Proclined maxillary anterior teeth

## Step 10.1 Immediate Dentures

### Advantage of Both Techniques

- Single tray technique: Ease of handling, if tissue undercuts are minimal to ensure satisfactory peripheral extensions
- Double tray technique: Stable index/joint between the 1st and the 2nd tray results in acceptable definitive impressions.

## Maxillomandibular Relationship

Due to advanced periodontal condition, migrated teeth result in loss of vertical dimension and change in occlusal plane. This needs to be assessed before recording jaw relation. Several methods are combined to determine the correct VDO such as, esthetics and phonetics, rest position evaluation and Niswonger's method.

In patients with multiple remaining teeth the centric relation is recorded at the finalized vertical dimension with the help of bite registration wax or other bite registration materials **(Fig. 10.1.14)**

In case, only anterior teeth are present, wax rims are made for recording the centric relation similar to conventional denture cases. **(Fig. 10.1.15)**

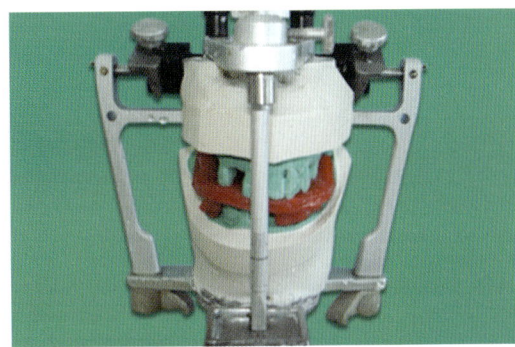

Fig. 10.1.14: Centric relation recorded and transferred to the articulator

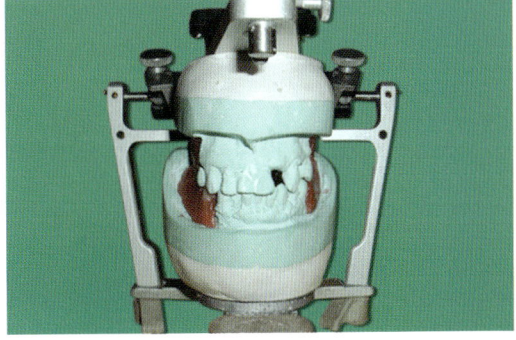

Fig. 10.1.15: In absence of posterior teeth, occlusal wax rims are utilized to record the centric relation and then transferred to the articulator

## Selection, Arrangement and Trial

Clinician must transfer the facial midline, canine lines, the plane of occlusion to the cast for the technician to visualize and change what needs to be corrected in the final denture **(Fig. 10.1.16)**. The shape, size, position and colour can be mimicked from the remaining teeth if desired by the patient.

Initially the missing teeth are arranged and a trial done in the patients mouth. Again the changes are noted and marked if possible for the corrections in the immediate dentures **(Fig. 10.1.17)**.

## Teeth Placement

Removal of natural teeth on the stone cast and placement of denture teeth:
- Teeth are removed to the level of the gingival margin **(Fig. 10.1.18)**
- Socket depth should be limited ideally to 5 mm labially following the long axis of the tooth. Socket is shaped in a convex form
- Edges are rounded, smoothened after trimming

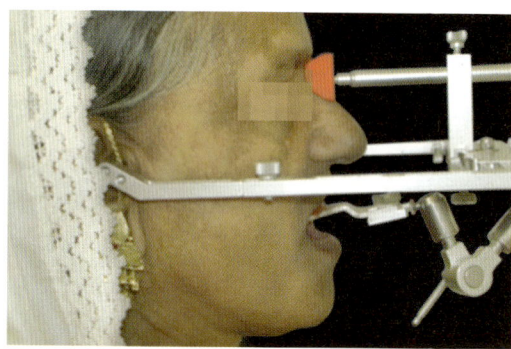

Fig. 10.1.16: Facebow can be used to transfer the occlusal plane and other parameters to the articulator

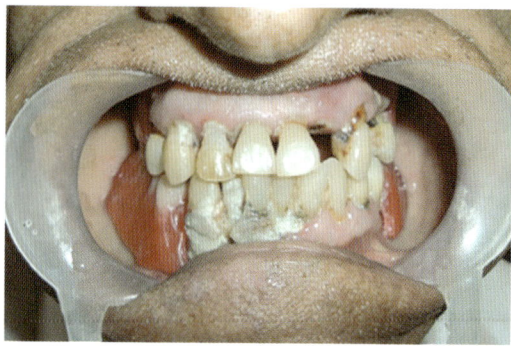

Fig. 10.1.17: Try in done and the corrections made

## Periodontal Probing

The depths of the pockets around natural teeth need to be evaluated and the amount of reduction/preparation of the cast be mentioned to the laboratory technician. A clinical probing helps to prevent under/over contouring of the sockets.

## Surgical Template Fabrication

- A trimmed duplicate cast is poured
- A clear acrylic template is fabricated: This template will be utilized as a guide during extractions to ensure all bony undercuts are removed during surgery **(Fig. 10.1.19)**
- If the anterior teeth are in the correct place and the patient desires the placement/position of the teeth to be maintained in the immediate denture then a labial/palatal index is made before trimming the teeth off
- This index can be utilized to place teeth in the original pre extraction position **(Figs 10.1.20 and 10.1.21)**.

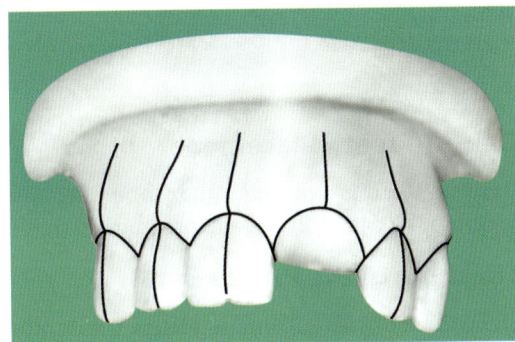

Fig. 10.1.18: Tooth removal to the level of gingival margin

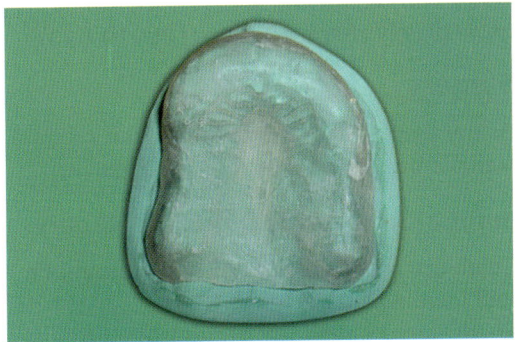

Fig. 10.1.19: Fabrication of clear acrylic template to ensure removal of all bony spicules and undercuts during surgery

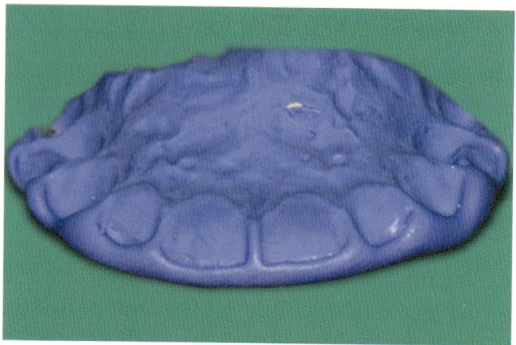

**Fig. 10.1.20:** Palatal index to record the position of the original anterior teeth prior to extraction

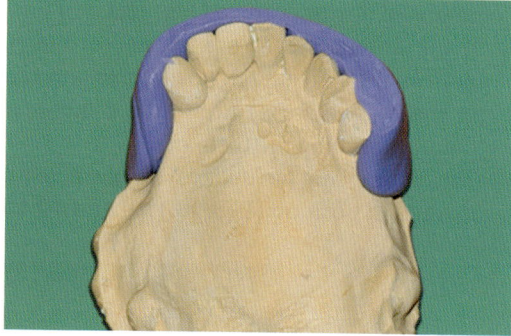

**Fig. 10.1.21:** Labial index helps is record and eventually mimic (if desired by the patient) the labio-palatal relation of the remaining natural anterior teeth

## Denture Teeth Placement

Denture teeth are placed one by one after trimming the remaining teeth on the cast utilizing the pre marked parameters **(Fig. 10.1.22)**.

## Finishing of the Prosthesis

Once the teeth arrangement is done the denture is flasked, dewaxed and acrylized. After finishing and polishing, it is ready to be delivered immediately after extractions **(Fig. 10.1.23)**.

## Surgery

As there are multiple extractions, the surgical procedure should be well planned and explained to the patient.

### Surgical Steps on the Day of the Surgery

Teeth are removed carefully maintaining the integrity of the labial and lingual plates **(Fig. 10.1.24)**.
- Regional blocks are administered to avoid tissue distortion by local infiltrations

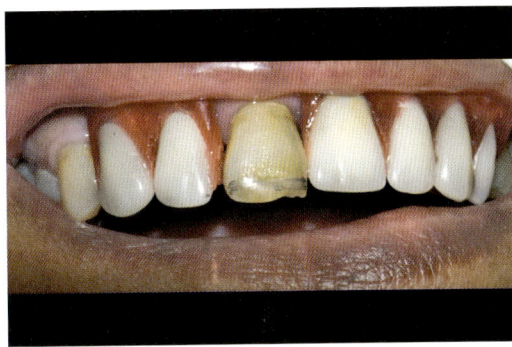

**Fig. 10.1.22:** Remaining natural teeth are removed one by one and replaced by denture teeth after the marked parameters are considered

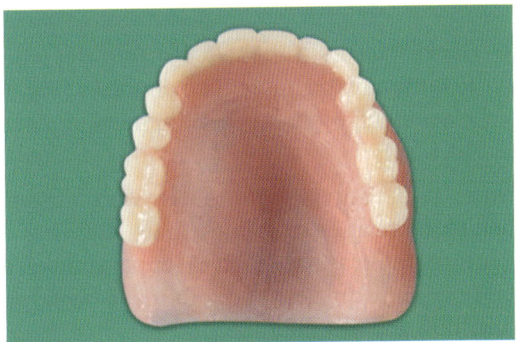

**Fig. 10.1.23:** Finished maxillary denture

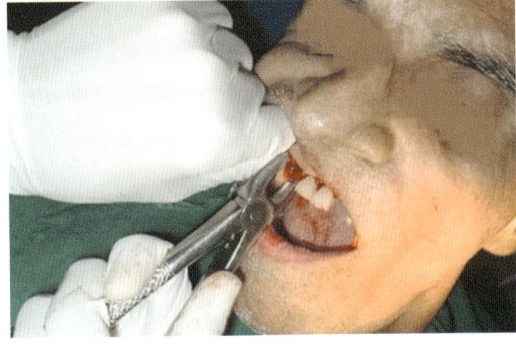

**Fig. 10.1.24:** Integrity of the labial and lingual plates is maintained during extraction phase

- Teeth are removed with minimal soft and hard tissue trauma **(Fig. 10.1.25)**
- Insertion of the surgical template to ascertain areas requiring minor alveoplasty
- These areas will show tissue blanching on compression of the template through the clear acrylic base **(Fig. 10.1.26)**
- Elimination of bony prominences in the areas of blanching to ensure denture stability

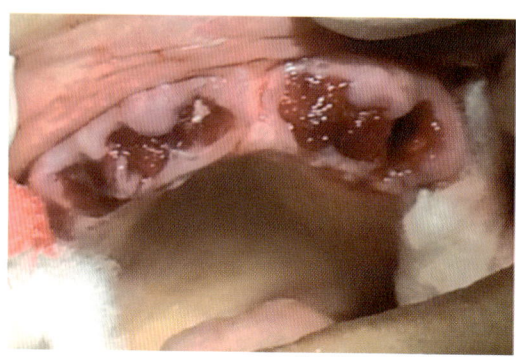

Fig. 10.1.25: Minimal hard and soft tissue trauma during extraction seen

- Socket closure with the help of sutures when required
- Insertion of the immediate dentures **(Fig. 10.1.27)**
- Placement of tissue conditioners if deemed necessary **(Fig. 10.1.28)**.

**Note:** If patient is comfortable with posterior teeth extractions before fabricating the immediate dentures then, there is a pre denture fabrication surgical appointment and a post denture fabrication extraction appointment with simultaneous denture insertion appointment.

## ■ INSERTION TIMELINE

**Flowchart:** This is an approximate insertion time line which is subject to change according to various factors, such as number of teeth present, extent and location of soft and hard tissue undercuts and patient compliance

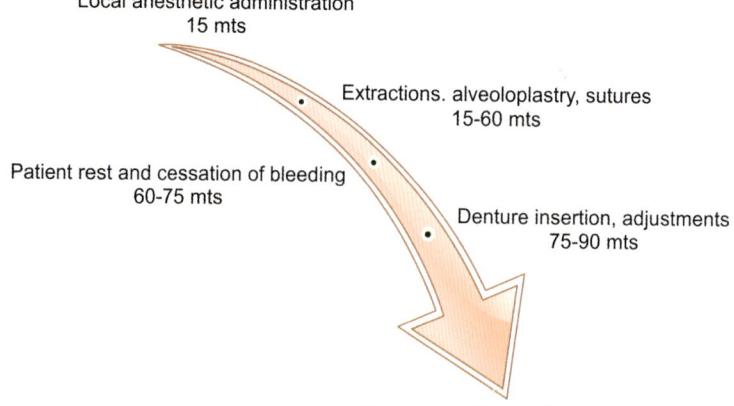

Local anesthetic administration
15 mts

Extractions. alveoloplastry, sutures
15-60 mts

Patient rest and cessation of bleeding
60-75 mts

Denture insertion, adjustments
75-90 mts

Tissue conditioners if required
90-120 mts

## Step 10.1 Immediate Dentures

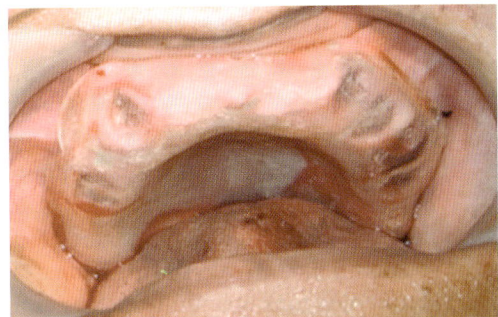

Fig. 10.1.26: Placement of clear acrylic template in the maxilla immediately after extractions to check for blanching to assess areas of compression

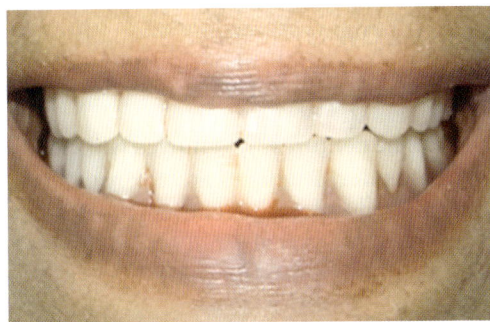

Fig. 10.1.27: Denture insertion immediately after extractions: Centric relation checked

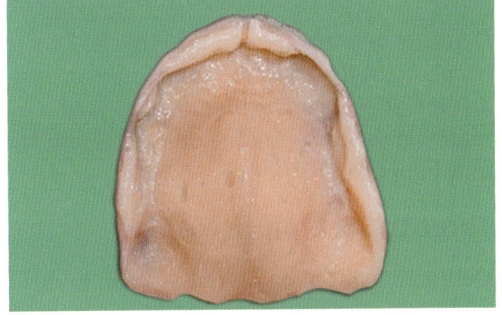

Fig. 10.1.28: Placement of tissue conditioner on the impression surface if needed

## POST INSERTION CARE

- It is advisable not to remove the immediate dentures for 24 hours as the dentures may not fit again after removal, due to post extraction tissue swelling
- Minor occlusal discrepancies may be present at the time of insertion due to interferences in occlusion. These should be addressed before sending the patient home as will cause tissue irritation, resulting in prolonged healing and loss of denture retention.

## PATIENT INSTRUCTIONS

- Do not remove the dentures for 24 hours
- Clinician will remove the dentures after 24 hours at tomorrow's next appointment
- If it comes lose, please put it back immediately and try to keep it in place
- Soft or liquid diet to be administered for 24 hours
- Avoid spitting and even rinsing in an exaggerated manner
- Take medications including analgesics as prescribed.

## FOLLOW UP

### 24 Hours Visit

Immediate dentures are removed with delicacy as the extraction sites will be tender. Dentures are cleansed and checked for sore spots. Once the sore spots are relieved, the denture is checked for the fit. If a tissue conditioner was not placed during insertion appointment it may be placed now depending on the patient's need.

### One / Two Week Visit

Denture bearing tissues are checked for presence of sore spots which are relieved in the immediate dentures. Occlusion is refined further. Socket convexities on the intaglio surface of the denture are removed to prevent tissue defects. Application of tissue conditioner may be repeated.

### Three to Six Months Visit

Dentures will need a reline due to loss of adaptation to the underlying denture base area. Permanent soft reline can be utilized to refit the dentures at this stage. A new set of dentures can now be fabricated if required as the frequency of bone loss is reduced and denture bearing tissues are stable.

## ADVANTAGES

- Patients are more comfortable with extractions once they are assured that they will not be without teeth at any time in public. This helps the patient psychologically and allows them to continue with their daily life without any hindrance

## Step 10.1 Immediate Dentures

- As the prosthesis is inserted immediately after the extractions, patient's appearance does not have any discernable change. Circum oral support ie: Muscle tone is maintained along with the lips and cheek fullness
- Unfavorable speech patterns can be avoided as the teeth can be placed in the same position as the natural ones
- Immediate denture also acts a bandage/splint over the extraction sockets as it covers the wound. By keeping food particles and any external irritants away from the site the prosthesis also helps in controlling the bleeding, ensuring the blood clot stays in place resulting in faster healing and less pain
- Mastication and the digestive functions are not hampered as teeth are always present. The diet is limited after placement of the immediate dentures till the patient gets used to the appliance
- Easier compliance and adaptability as the patient is very conscious about being edentulous
- Spreading out of the tongue and masticatory muscle enlargement can be controlled
- Residual ridges are subject to less resorption as immediate loading helps in maintaining a balance between the osteoblastic and osteoclastic activity resulting in healthy, well preserved ridges
- Better long term stability of the relined immediate prosthesis or the permanent prosthesis due to less resorption of the ridges as they are loaded early
- Remaining natural teeth may act as a guide to help in replicating the shape, size, colour and arrangement of the denture teeth.

## ■ DISADVANTAGES

- The major disadvantage of an immediate denture prosthesis is that it will not last long. As the bone under the dentures will resorb and remodel at a fast rate, the dentures will become lose soon. Either several relines have to be done or finally a new set of dentures be fabricated once the resorption is reduced and the base area has stabilized
- More appointments are required especially for adjustments and relines

- Usually the patients try to maintain their natural anterior teeth till the last minute. The immediate dentures cannot have an anterior trial before final insertion. Therefore, the esthetic outcome cannot be evaluated or ascertained
- Procedure is precise and time consuming needing more appointments making the treatment expensive compared to a conventional complete denture
- **Challenging:** Due to the presence of natural teeth, bony undercuts (anterior maxilla) and areas of edentulous pockets, it is difficult to determine the correct relations and to record good impressions.

## Conclusion

- A thorough medical history is to be evaluated and a clinical, diagnostic and radiographic examination is done to understand the extent of bone loss of remaining teeth.
- Immediate denture fabrication requires multiple extractions, long appointments, superior clinical skills, abundant patient compliance and an increase in the total treatment cost.
- Patient should be made aware about the bone resorption process after extractions and the chances of dentures becoming lose gradually.
- Dentures will have to be adjusted, relined and eventually remade if required depending on the amount of bone resorption.

# Step 10.2

## Relining Procedures

*"The softest things in the world overcome the hardest things in the world"*

*Lao Tzu*

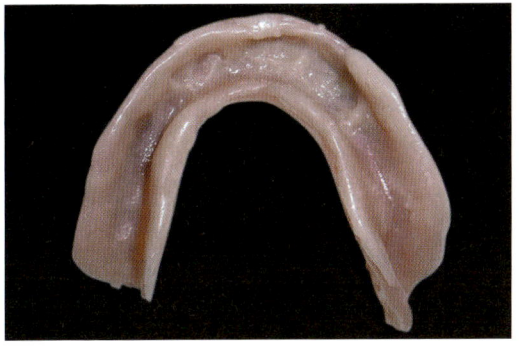

# Step 10.2

# Relining Procedures

## ■ INTRODUCTION

Complete denture as a treatment modality requires diligent patient maintenance and intermittent dental office visits to check for denture fit and signs of changes in the denture-bearing areas.

Denture base adaptation to the underlying hard and soft tissues is important and needs monitoring via regular recall schedule. The magnitude of discrepancies developed as a result of prosthesis wear and/or changes in the denture-bearing areas with time and age determines the need for reline, rebase or a remake of the denture **(Fig. 10.2.1)**.

## ■ OBSERVED CLINICAL CHANGES

- Lose dentures: Loss of retention and stability
- Reduced vertical dimension: Occlusal wear

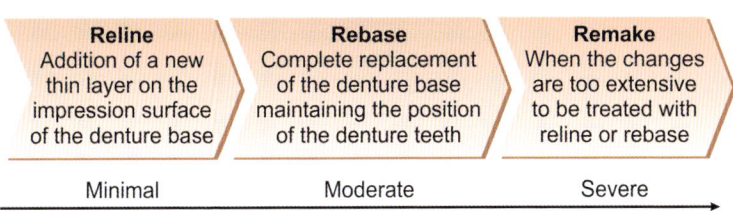

**Fig. 10.2.1:** Discrepancies developed due to denture wear in a long time denture wearer

- Horizontal shift of dentures: Attrition **(Fig. 10.2.2)** resulting in incorrect centric relation **(Fig. 10.2.3)**
- Loss of facial tissue support: Older looking appearance, drooping of line angles **(Fig. 10.2.4)**
- Occlusal plane discrepancy
- Cracks, stains and fractures.

Long-span denture wearers often complain of lose dentures, inefficient mastication, soreness of the oral tissues, unacceptable esthetics and in severe cases even pain, dribbling of saliva from the corners of the mouth, hyperplasia and redness of the denture-bearing tissues **(Fig. 10.2.5)**.

It is imperative to understand the cause of changes and the severity. The cause maybe an unharmonious occlusion due to denture wear or changes in the oral tissues.

Once the problems are diagnosed, an appropriate treatment plan can be formulated.

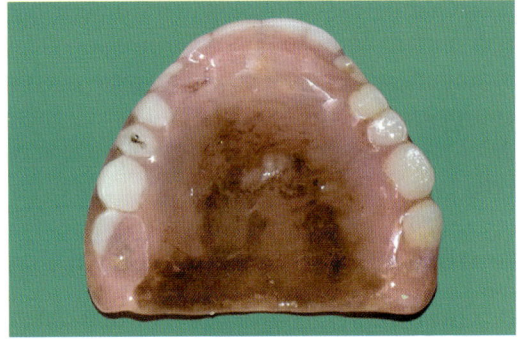

Fig. 10.2.2: Discrepancies developed as a result of prosthesis wear

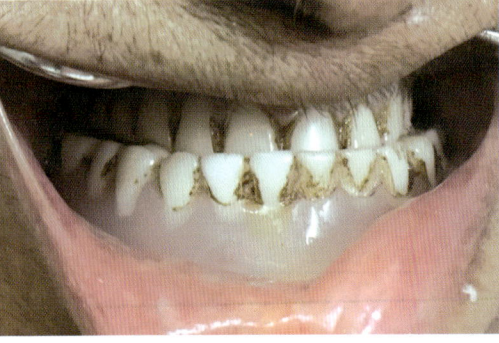

Fig. 10.2.3: Denture wear causing Horizontal shift of mandible leading to a pseudo class III jaw relation

## Step 10.2 Relining Procedures

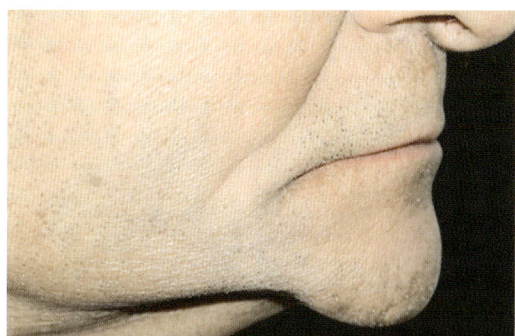

Fig. 10.2.4: Loss of facial tissue support due to change in vertical dimension leading to older looking appearance and drooping of line angles

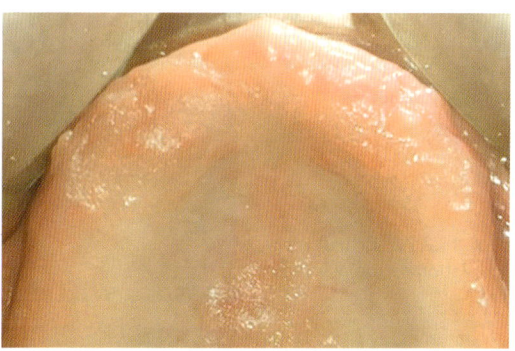

Fig. 10.2.5: Denture Hyperplasia: Inflamed denture bearing area

### ■ CHECKS TO REACH THE CORRECT DIAGNOSIS

- Independent assessment of the denture bases to check the stability and retention without occlusal influence/interference. Anteroposterior-lateral movement will be limited to a mere 1–2 mm in stable denture bases
- Rocking during vertical loading
- Clinical evaluation: Presence of inflamed or hyperplastic tissue
- Prognathic mandible: Forward rotational movement of the jaw due to loss of vertical dimension
- Examination of the patient's frontal face, profile including the lips, facial angles, chin to nose distance **(Fig. 10.2.6)**
- Observe the occlusal plane in relation to the ala-tragus **(Fig. 10.2.7)**, smile line in relation to the interpupillary line for esthetics **(Fig. 10.2.8)**
- Observe which ridge has resorbed more or has been uniform to understand the interarch occlusal harmony **(Fig. 10.2.9)**.

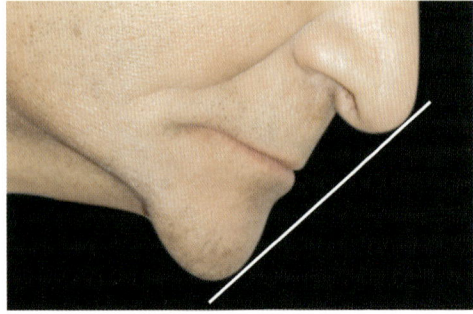

**Fig. 10.2.6:** Patient wearing newly fabricated complete dentures. Observe satisfactorily restored nose to chin distance

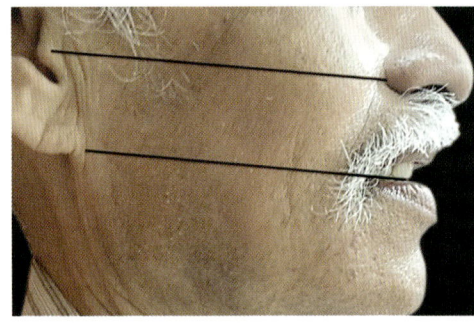

**Fig. 10.2.7:** Occlusal plane in relation to the ala-tragus line

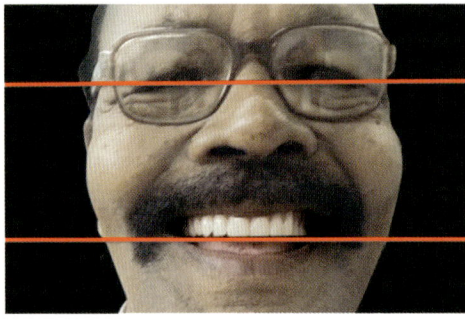

**Fig. 10.2.8:** Smile line in relation to the interpupillary line for a pleasant appearance

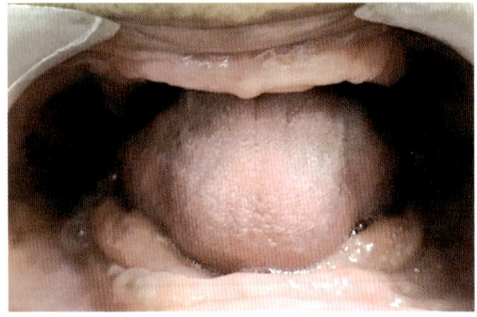

**Fig. 10.2.9:** Both the ridges have to be observed in relation to each other ie: resorption patterns have to be analyzed to assess the interarch occlusal harmony

## Hyperplastic Inflamed Tissues

As a pretreatment plan, it is a must to reduce and eventually eliminate the inflammation and consequently the hyperplastic tissues to normal before a treatment is started.

Ideally, the patient is asked to not wear the dentures for 24–48 hours to ensure healing. During this time period, the inflamed tissue recovers and normalizes. The denture fit and relations are re-evaluated with the use of pressure indicating paste (PIP).

## Alternative Method

Most of the patients agree to keep the dentures out of the oral cavity for the time period requested by the dentist for healing to occur. Some patients are not comfortable without the dentures. They refuse to be without the dentures even for a day. One must understand patient apprehensions and respect their views and demands.

In these instances, the clinician can apply a soft tissue conditioner for 2–3 days and the tissues re evaluated in the next visit. Applying the tissue conditioner helps in healing without forcing the patients to be edentulous even for a day helping them to continue with their social life unhampered.

Patient should be informed that after the tissue conditioner application the fit of the dentures will improve and the dentures will feel more comfortable for some time. It is a temporary, transient treatment as the material is subject to deformation thus necessitating the need for a permanent treatment at a later stage **(Fig. 10.2.10)**.

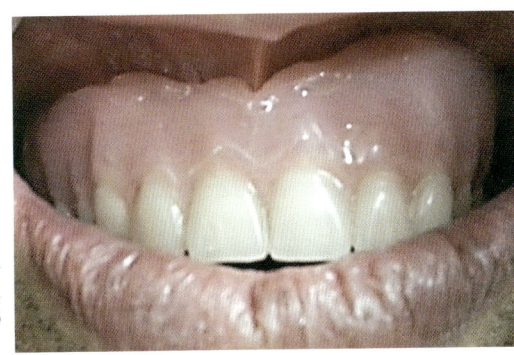

Fig. 10.2.10: Tissue conditioner as temporary, transient treatment to enhance patient comfort

Impression making for relining or rebasing is similar and is a technique sensitive procedure. Suggested impression procedures for relining are as follows:
- Open mouth technique
- Closed mouth technique
- Combination technique
- Dynamic technique/functional impression technique.

Any technique employed to get acceptable results needs some basic preparation. One must ensure that the tissue undercuts are minimal in reline or rebase cases. Clinical stages of tissue conditioners are depicted in **Table 10.2.1** and denture and tissue preparation is described in **Table 10.2.2**.

Table 10.2.1: **Stages of tissue conditioners after application**

| Plostic Stage | Elastic Stage | Final Stage |
| --- | --- | --- |
| • Immediately after application to few hours<br>• Fit is improved, reduced occlusal stresses | • Few hours to 3-7 days after application<br>• Slight hardening of the material<br>• Reduction in occlusal stresses along with fit is still maintained | • 1-2 weeks after application<br>• Firm, hard surface<br>• Reduction in fit and occlusal disharmony<br>• Surface deteriorating with time |

Table 10.2.2: **Tissue and denture preparation**

| Tissue Preparation | Denture Preparation |
| --- | --- |
| Abused mucosa must be allowed to heal by either keeping the dentures out or by application of tissue conditioners | An even amount 2 mm of impression surface of the denture is to be removed (**Fig. 10.2.11**) |
| Excessive hypertrophic tissues/epulis in the denture-bearing area should be excised surgically | Denture surface is cleansed of the debris |
| Massage the denture-bearing area with the pad of the index finger/soft brush to improve blood circulation | Occlusion is perfected with the help of minor selective grinding |
| Removal of severe tissue undercuts, developed with time | Check the denture borders and grind accordingly as the dentures will be used as trays to remake the final accurate impression surface |

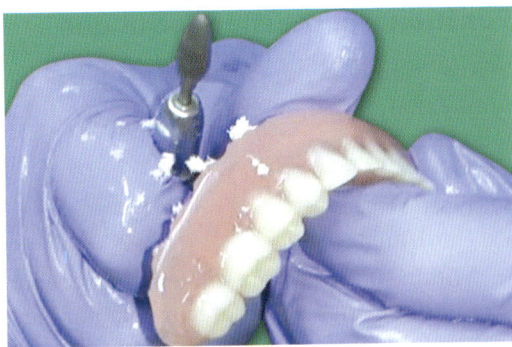

Fig. 10.2.11: An even amount of denture surface (2mm) is removed

## CLINICAL IMPRESSION PROCEDURES

### Open Mouth Technique

Each impression, maxillary and mandibular is made separately. The old dentures are used as trays. Border molding is done with tissue stops to help reorient the border molded dentures again for the placement for final impression making. Movements are done similar to the border molding during new denture fabrication. Minor occlusal discrepancies are corrected either directly in the oral cavity or with a laboratory remount.

### Closed Mouth Technique

In this procedure as well, the dentures are used as custom trays. The border molding is done by the patient and the dentures are held/oriented in the mouth by occluding with the opposing denture. This technique is used once the basic occlusion is corrected prior to impression making.

### Combination Technique

It is a combination of both open and closed mouth techniques. Most commonly used relining/rebasing impression technique. It is important to ensure that the occlusion is perfected and large undercuts relieved before beginning. Here, the border molding material is molded in the oral cavity by the clinician initially, after which the patient is asked to occlude against the opposite arch denture for orientation. Patient molds the peripheries further in a closed position by puckering and smiling.

## Functional Impression Technique

Tissue conditioners/temporary soft liners have also been used as impression materials. These go through three stages which are as follows:
- Plastic stage
- Elastic stage
- Hard/final stage.

Within 10-15 days the soft temporary relines reach a firm or hard stage, i.e. the impressions are now stable. These impressions are sent to the laboratory for a remount and further processing of the dentures. This is a completely physiological reline as all the movements are done by the patient over time. As this material does not create sufficient displacement of soft tissues in the posterior palatal seal (PPS) area, it needs to either be built with another material or the area scraped in the cast to form a seal. Studies demonstrate that this procedure is as successful as others if used with caution.

## Permanent Soft Reline Materials

Currently, newer reline materials by various companies have made their presence felt as they claim that their soft reline lasts for a minimum of 18-24 months without getting stained or the material peeling away from the dentures. A form of combination technique is used, as these materials set in the oral cavity within 5-7 minutes as mentioned by the manufacturer. Once completely set they do not change color or form for a long time making them materials of choice where a hard reline is not suggested **(Fig. 10.2.12)**.

Ideally, the lower denture must be relined first and made stable before the upper is relined. Due to the lesser surface area for the lower denture, chances of mandibular denture instability are more and thus need to be stabilized first.

Excess material can be removed by cutting with a Bard-Parker (BP) blade and some areas may need a sharp scissor. The junction of the reline and the hard acrylic denture can be smoothened with the help of pre and high polish silicon points **(Fig. 10.2.13)**.

Potential problems associated with soft, resilient liners:
- Potential for abuse **(Fig. 10.2.14)**
- Unequal pressure may result in uneven material placement leading to unstable dentures

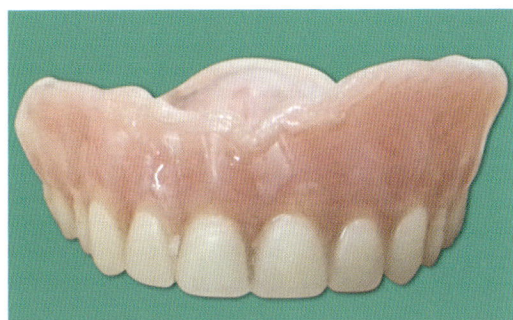

Fig. 10.2.12: Manufacturer's claim varying time period of sustainability (approx 6months to 2years) of the permanent chairside relines

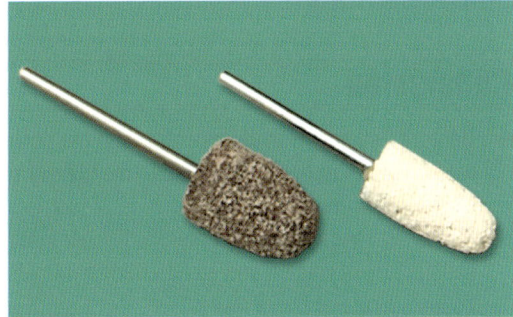

Fig. 10.2.13: Pre and high polish silicon points to adjust the soft relines and merge the liner and the denture borders

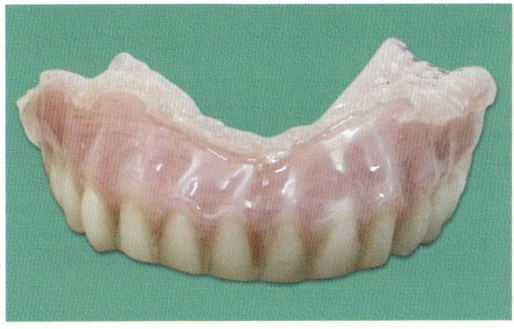

Fig. 10.2.14: Peeling of soft liner, showing porosities

- Occlusal discrepancies
- Excessive increase in vertical dimension
- Loss of denture orientation/change in plane of occlusion
- Possible alteration in facial support.

These materials are direct application, chair-side relines which give immediate results. Hard/soft reline materials which are sent to the laboratory for processing, finishing, polishing are called Indirect application relines **(Fig. 10.2.15)**.

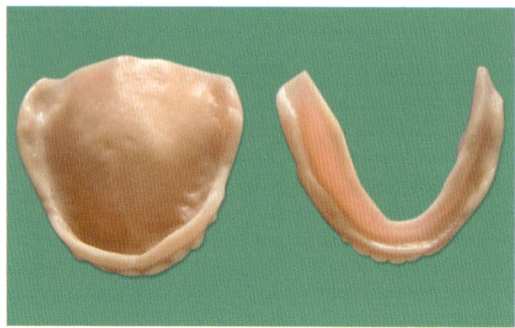

Fig. 10.2.15: Permanent laboratory processed soft reline

## Conclusion

- Denture Relining procedures come with their own pros and cons. Though many such materials are available, the clinical procedure for all remains almost the same.
- Reline is recommended only if the dentures to be relined have a satisfactory occlusion and all other key parameters are acceptable except tissue surface of the dentures.
- Relines help to improve denture base adaptation to the underlying denture bearing tissues resulting in improved denture retention and stability.

# Step 10.3

## Denture Repairs

*"It is the neglect of timely repair that makes rebuilding necessary"*
Richard Whately

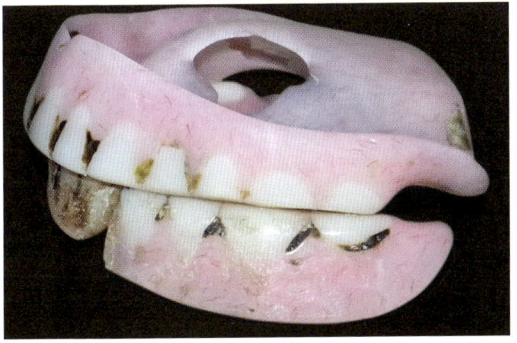

# Step 10.3

# Denture Repairs

## INTRODUCTION

Dentures can fracture and may need repair. Two common reasons for fracture are:
1. Fall / patient dropped the dentures
2. Malfunction:
   - Incorrect occlusion
   - Fulcrum creation due to unstable / improper / warped dentures
   - Chewing forces on the denture
   - Material used in denture fabrication.

Denture fall is the most common cause of fracture in complete dentures. Due to the unavailability of the doctor at that precise moment along with the functional and psychological discomfort the patient faces due to inability to wear the dentures results in panic. Many a times, such patients try to "fix" the dentures on their own resulting in loss of the marginal integrity of the denture base, thus magnifying a small problem many fold. Often such dentures become unfit for repair and may need to be refabricated from the scratch.

If the fracture pieces do not approximate completely, it is advisable to re fabricate the denture as the chances of success are bleak.

## Types of Denture Fractures

- Midline Fractures **(Fig. 10.3.1)**
- Tooth Fractures:
  - Single tooth fracture **(Fig. 10.3.2)**
  - Multiple tooth fracture

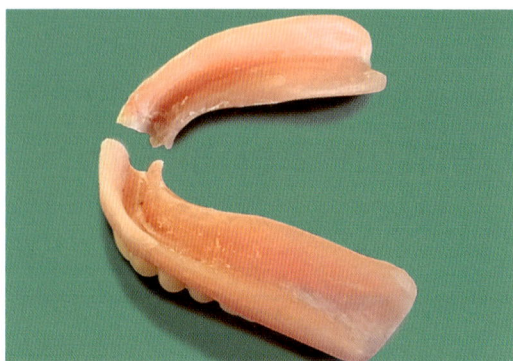

Fig. 10.3.1: Midline fracture of a mandibular denture

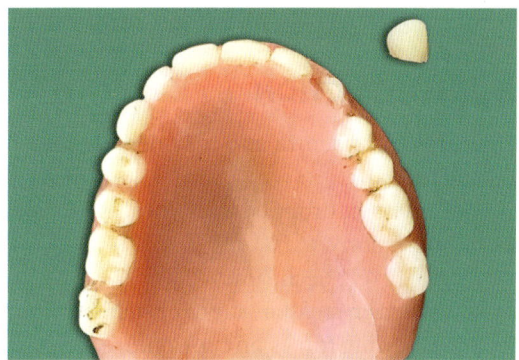

Fig. 10.3.2: Single tooth fracture

- Denture base fractures:
    - One or more small parts that can be aligned
    - Small fractured part: Missing.

Large fracture repairs are advisable to be done in the laboratory as the process is time consuming for the dentist and needs more precision than a small repair which may be done chair side.

## Types of Repairs

| Type | Disadvantage |
| --- | --- |
| Cold cure/Self cure | Lack of strength and colour instability |
| Heat cure | May cause denture warpage |
| Light cure | Lack of strength, additional curing unit cost |

## Basic Repair Procedure

- Fractured pieces are approximated and checked for accurate fit. **(Figs 10.3.3 and 10.3.4)**
- The assembled pieces are held together with sticky wax
- An index is made by:
  - Pouring plaster after blocking undercuts as/if needed
  - Packing hard laboratory silicon in the under surface **(Figs 10.3.5 to 10.3.7)**.
- The repaired denture is removed from the index and cleansed of sticky wax
- 2-3mm of the acrylic is removed from the fractured segment edges to give a bevel. A long, deep and rounded bevel is created along the outer surface of the denture pieces **(Fig. 10.3.8)**
- The beveled pieces are placed back on the index. A separating medium is applied if a plaster cast has been poured. A silicon index does not stick to the repair acrylic and is much easier to handle

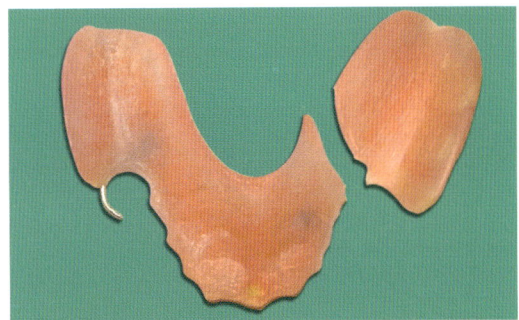

Fig. 10.3.3: Fractured pieces are approximated and checked for accurate fit

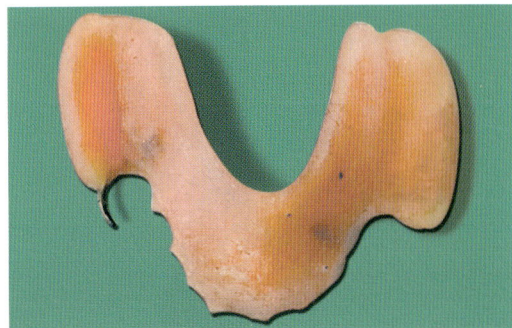

Fig. 10.3.4: Repaired denture

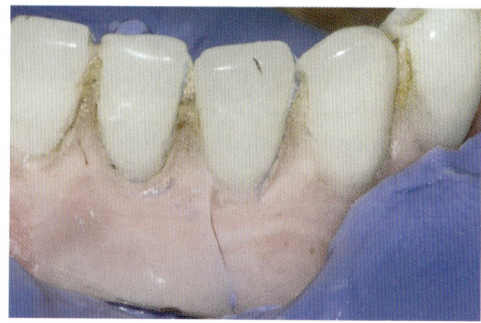

**Fig. 10.3.5:** Hard laboratory silicon in the under surface: Fracture line

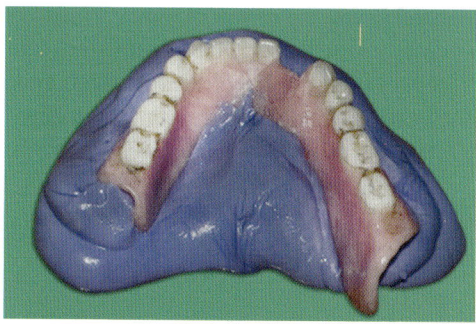

**Fig. 10.3.6:** Hard silicon is packed in place of plaster

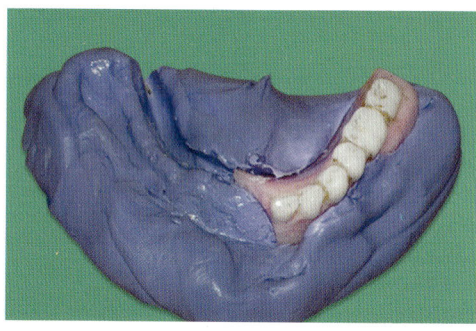

**Fig. 10.3.7:** Denture parts are removed and replaced to ensure proper alignment and approximation of the fractured denture

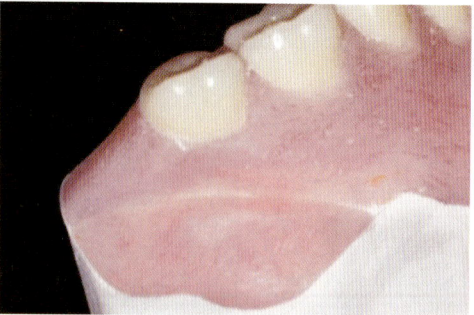

**Fig. 10.3.8:** Rounded bevel is created along the outer surface of the denture pieces to increase surface area for bonding and also to mask the fracture line

## Step 10.3 Denture Repairs

- Wet or pre moisturize the beveled areas with monomer using a brush to place and remove excess
- Mix adequate monomer polymer in a dappen dish. As a thin, flow consistency is achieved, small increments are placed and smoothened simultaneously with a paint brush
- Once filled, the prosthesis is kept in a pressure pot for approximately 30 minutes at 30pps pressure submerged under 100 degree F water to increase the repair strength
- The repaired denture is removed from the index and finishing done with acrylic burs and stones
- Polishing is completed with pumice and wheel.

## An Alternate Method

Another method for chair side repair uses light cure repair material:
- A thin coating of light cure bond is applied on the beveled surfaces
- A small piece of light cure material is cut and rolled to the desired shape
- This material is packed / pressed into the beveled fractured line area
- The material is blended with the help of repair liquid and a brush to merge into its surrounding surfaces
- The area must be coated with an oxy air barrier before placement into the light curing unit
- An intense visible light in the 400-500-nm range for 10-15 minutes is required for complete curing to occur
- The cured repair requires minimal finishing and polishing.

**Advantages**

Its advantages over conventional self-cure resins is mentioned in **Flowchart 10.3.1**.

**Flowchart 10.3.1:** Advantages of using light-cure repair material over conventional self-cure resins

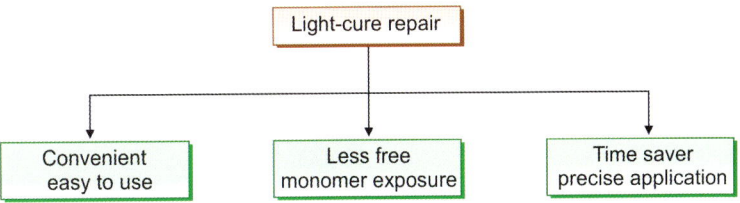

## Denture Base Strengtheners

Sometimes only acrylic in dentures is not enough. Few patient's may exert great masticatory pressure while chewing. In such cases the dentures can get fractured while chewing within the oral cavity. This is more commonly seen when one arch has acrylic denture opposing natural teeth. Natural teeth occluding against dentures may create unnatural and extremely heavy masticatory forces resulting in midline fractures.

Such dentures require strengtheners with in the denture bases. Complete metal bases or smaller metal parts in the denture base can be used as strengtheners where as denture borders are of acrylic in entirety. Metals most commonly used are:
- Cobalt chromium cast strengthener
- Stainless steel
- Aluminium.

In literature, gold has also been used as a strengthener under acrylic dentures.

## Fractured Tooth Repair

As an emergency procedure, a small portion of a fractured tooth can be repaired with free hand composite and the patient can take the dentures home in no time **(Figs 10.3.9 and 10.3.10)**.

For larger fractures or multiple fractures, the fractured teeth have to be removed with an acrylic trimming bur along with some of the surrounding acrylic resin to create space for repair resin. Once the teeth/mold have been identified and matched with the remaining teeth, the slots are made ready. Before the tooth/teeth

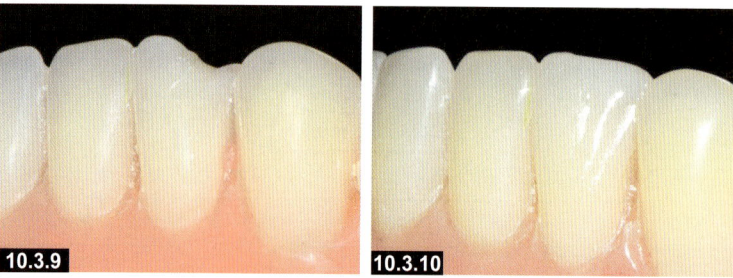

**Fig. 10.3.9:** Small portion of a fractured tooth. **Fig. 10.3.10:** Free hand repair with composite

## Step 10.3 Denture Repairs

are tacked in space and fixed with sticky wax to hold them in place, a groove is made on the lingual surface of the tooth. This groove helps in increasing adhesion of the replacement tooth to the underlying denture base by increasing surface area.

In a dappen dish autopolymerizing resin is mixed in a thin consistency. The resin is placed in small increments with the help of a brush and each increment smoothened. Once the space around the tooth is filled and the material sufficiently adapted the repair acrylic is allowed to set. After an initial set the denture is placed in warm water for sufficient curing. It also results in leaching of the excess/unwanted monomer. The denture is finished and polished with the routine protocol.

Every clinician one time or the other faces the problem of denture repair. This chapter provides a basic know how ensuring that the clinician can understand and deliver a chairside repaired denture in the operatory with ease.

## Conclusion

- Slipping and falling of dentures is the most common cause of denture fracture. Fractures while chewing though possible and seen in clinical practices are still a minority and should be treated only when the cause is diagnosed.
- In a fractured denture, repair is to be initiated only when the fractured pieces can be approximated completely without any gaps to ensure success.
- Small tooth repairs can be done chairside with composites within the operatory by the clinician.

# Step 10.4

## Copy Dentures

*"The dentist must know human psychology because the ability to understand the patient's mental processes is frequently the difference between the acceptance and the rejection of Complete Dentures"*
*Charles M Heartwell Jr*

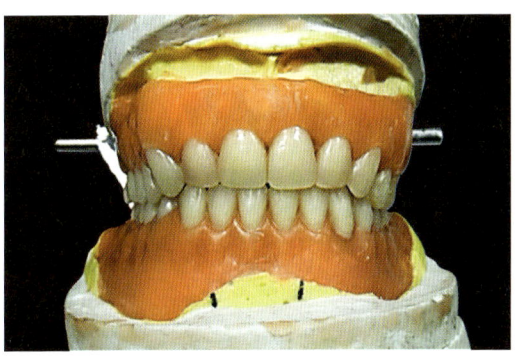

# Step 10.4

# Copy Dentures

## ■ REPLICA OR COPY DENTURE TECHNIQUE

At an advanced age, it is extremely difficult to adapt to change. It has been observed that geriatric patients wearing dentures are extremely vary when it comes to getting a new pair of dentures made. Many a times, they go on using old, misshapen and functionally inept dentures out of fear of getting new ones fabricated **(Figs 10.4.1A and B)**.

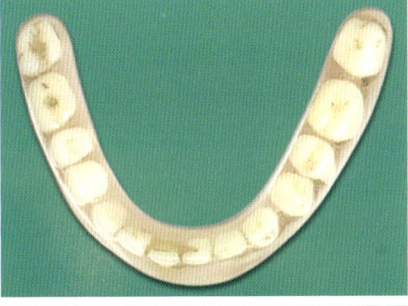

**Fig. 10.4.1A:** 30 years old functionally inept mandibular denture

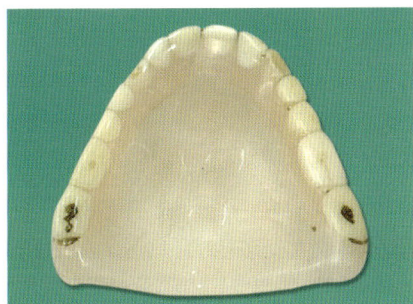

**Fig. 10.4.1B:** 30 years old maxillary denture: washed out appearance

**Common reason:** "The fear of inability to adjust to the new dentures".

An important element which has been identified in helping the patient to adjust to a new pair of complete dentures is to copy or replicate the shape of the polished surface.

With time, patient starts to utilize the orofacial musculature to keep the dentures in place. The replicated polished surface can help the patient to control and maneuver the new prosthesis with ease reducing difficulties associated with adaptation to a new denture.

In one of our denture wearing patients, a new denture was fabricated due to loss of vertical dimension or attrition in the old dentures. The increased surface area which was covered, vertical rehabilitation along with the change in the size and shape of the new complete denture prosthesis were evident on comparison **(Figs 10.4.2A and B)**.

Inspite of the improved function and esthetics the patient failed to adapt. He was more comfortable with the older functionally and esthetically compromised denture.

Therefore, in those cases where the clinician feels that the patient will not be able to adapt to the new dentures, the shape of the old dentures should be replicated. There are various factors which can be used to identify the patients who need duplicated dentures such as:
- Enlarged tongue
- Patient's age
- Patients with generalized neuromuscular deficit
- Reduced control due to diseases such as parkinsonism and stroke

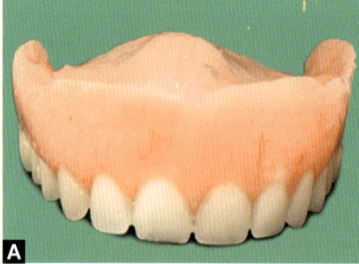 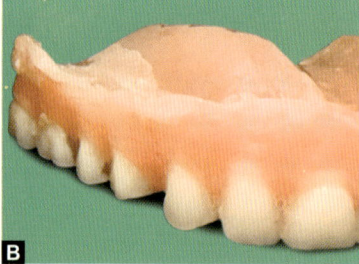

Figs 10.4.2A and B: New and old dentures of the same patient. Notice the new denture on the left is much larger than the existing old denture resulting in difficulty in adapting to the new prosthesis

- Condition of the old dentures
- Desire to have duplicate dentures.

There are various techniques that have been suggested and used over the years. In this chapter, denture duplicating techniques will be discussed along with their relevant variations.

## ■ COPY TECHNIQUE

**Purpose:** Replicating the shape of the polished surface of the old denture **(Fig. 10.4.3)**.

### Step by Step Procedure

- Recording the impressions of the existing dentures to produce replicas for the technician
- Intercuspal relation is recorded to help in mounting the replicas on the articulator
- Shade and mould of the existing teeth to either be replicated by the technician or changed, if needed on the clinician's instructions
- The replicas are tried in the mouth and checked for occlusion and overall esthetics
- Patients should be made aware that the replicas will be loose and the fit will be corrected at a later stage
- Once satisfied with the trial replicated dentures, definitive impressions are made
- A closed mouth impression technique is suggested or used in this procedure
- The position of the post dam must be marked with an indelible pencil on the maxillary impression to indicate the posterior extent of the denture

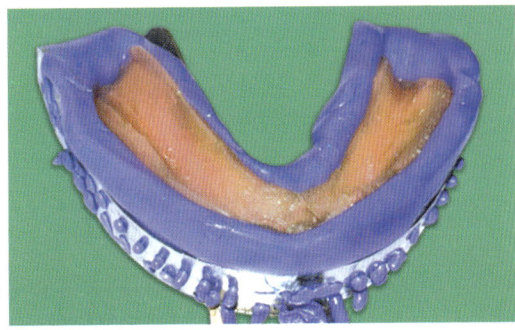

**Fig. 10.4.3:** Replicating the shape of the polished surface of the old denture with putty impression

- The dentures are processed and delivered to the patient with regular post insertion instructions.

There are various techniques in literature to record the impressions of the existing dentures. Below are few of the commonly used techniques **(Fig. 10.4.4)**.

## Soap Box Technique

- A plastic soap box is used with small cut out area for the sprues
- Alginate is filled on one-half of the box. The denture is placed with the occlusal surface embedded in the alginate (irreversible hydrocolloid)
- As the alginate sets, excess material is cut back to the box edge and petroleum jelly is applied on to the set alginate
- Alginate is mixed again, placed on the other half of the box and the soap box is closed tightly
- Excess material is removed and the box is placed on the counter to set
- Once set, the soap box is opened and the denture is removed.

## Double Metal Tray Technique

- A metal tray is loaded with alginate impression material and the old denture is embedded with the cameo surface inside the alginate until its flush with the material **(Figs 10.4.5A and B)**

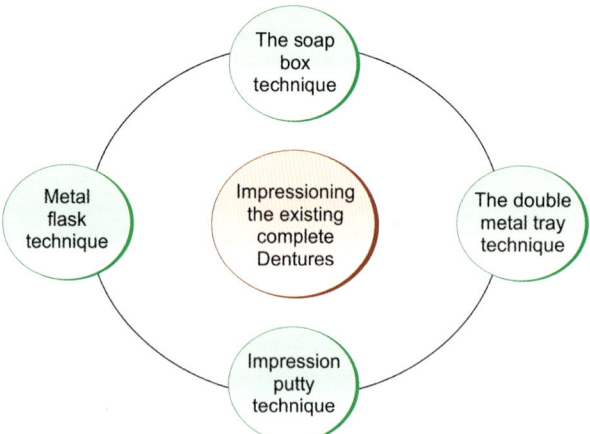

**Fig. 10.4.4:** Commonly used techniques to record the impressions of the existing dentures

## Step 10.4 Copy Dentures

- Once the alginate sets, three grooves are cut: one anteriorly and two buccally
- After placing the petroleum jelly, another tray is filled with alginate and inverted on top of the first tray recording the impression surface of the denture
- On setting, the dentures are removed from the trays and handed back to the patient **(Figs 10.4.6A and B)**.

### *Metal Flask Technique*

A metal flask used in a similar way has the advantage of being less flexible than the soap box technique and more predictable than the metal tray technique.

### *Impression Putty Technique*

This technique is a variant of double metal tray technique. The use of putty makes this a dimensionally more stable technique than the

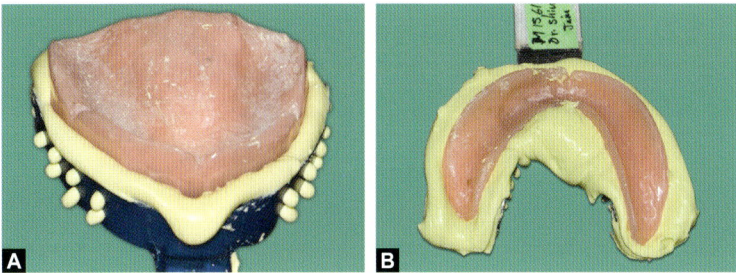

**Figs 10.4.5A and B:** Double metal tray technique: A metal tray is loaded with alginate impression material and the old denture is embedded with the occlusal surface inside the alginate until its flush with the material

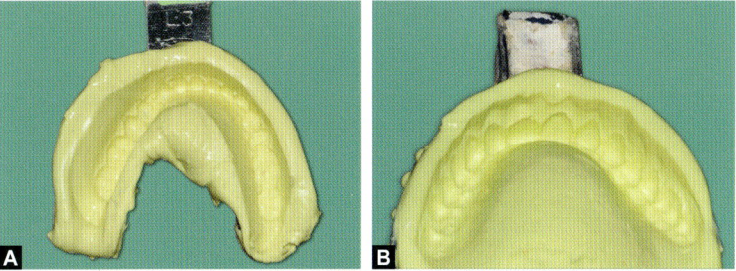

**Figs 10.4.6A and B:** After removing the dentures from the first set of alginate filled trays, anatomy and the polished surface of the dentures is recorded

alginate one especially if the technician delays making the replicas **(Figs 10.4.7A and B)**.

## Producing the Replicas

As the impressions are recorded, the dentist along with the technician decides the materials to be used in fabricating the replica, i.e. wax for the teeth and self-cured acrylic for the denture base.

### *Procedures*

- The molten wax is poured in the slots for teeth and as it sets, the remaining area is packed with cold cured acrylic **(Figs 10.4.8 and 10.4.9)**
- Sprues may be utilized for flowing the clear acrylic, completely filling the mold including the teeth and denture base
- The whole space for the material is filled with hardened wax, i.e.

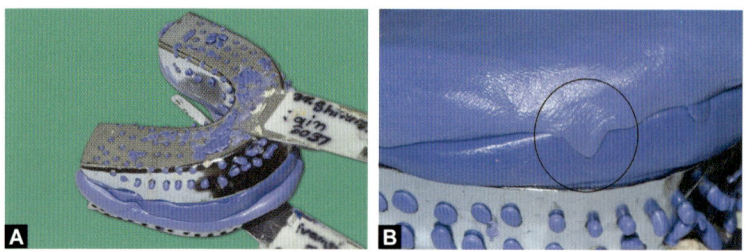

**Figs 10.4.7A and B:** Putty as a variant of double metal tray technique used with alginate. Three grooves are cut: one anteriorly and two buccally before placing the 2nd putty filled tray for orientation and to ensure proper seating

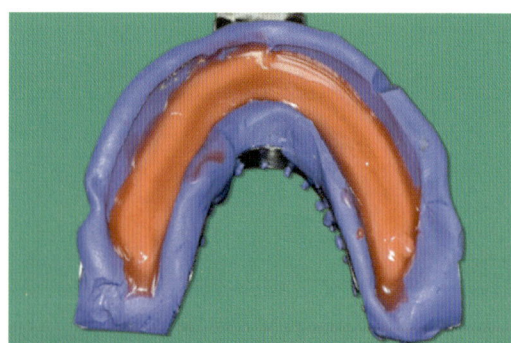

**Fig. 10.4.8:** The molten wax is poured in the slots for teeth

## Step 10.4 Copy Dentures

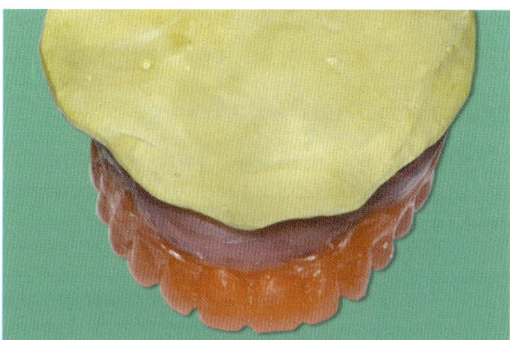

Fig. 10.4.9: Replicated maxillary teeth in wax

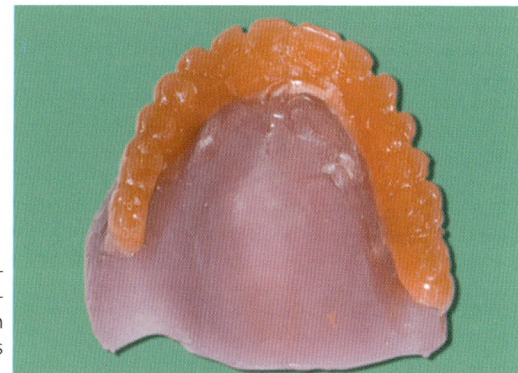

Fig. 10.4.10: Wax replicated teeth with the remaining area packed with light cured acrylic (in this case)

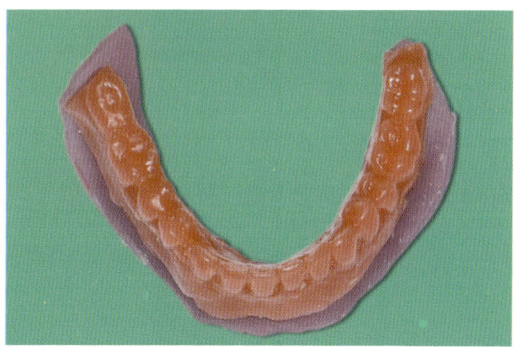

Fig. 10.4.11: Mandibular denture replica with wax teeth and acrylic base

"Hardened wax = Modelling wax + Sticky wax = Mixed together and poured" (**Figs 10.4.10 and 10.4.11**)

## Trial Dentures

Once the replicas have been mounted on an articulator with the help of the intercuspal bite material, the technician needs to discuss the tooth shade and mould with the dentist. If desired, the tooth shape and shade can be duplicated **(Figs 10.4.12 and 10.4.13)**.

## *Laboratory Trial Denture Stage*

Ideally, the wax teeth are removed individually and replaced by the appropriate acrylic teeth to get a completed trial denture **(Fig. 10.4.14)**.

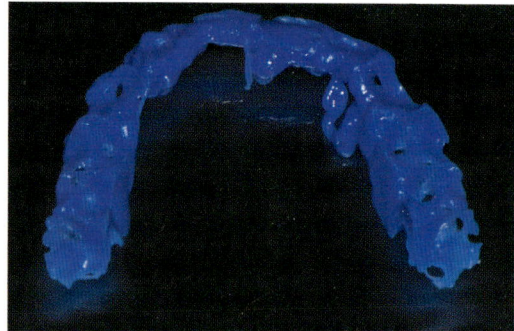

**Fig. 10.4.12:** Interocclusal bite material is used to mount the replicas on an articulator

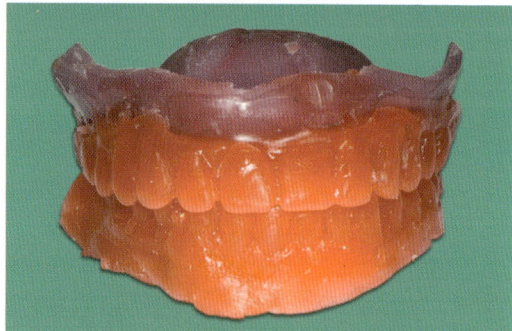

**Fig. 10.4.13:** Occlusal relation of the maxillary and mandibular replicas checked and then mounted

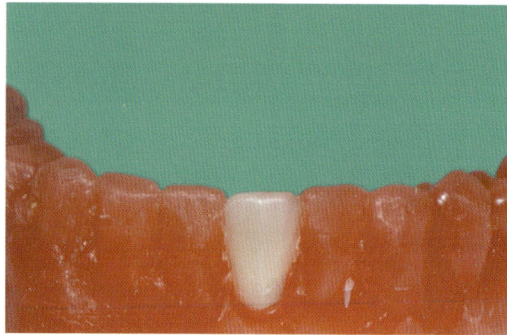

**Fig. 10.4.14:** The wax teeth are removed individually and replaced by the appropriate acrylic teeth

## Clinic Trial Denture Stage

The occlusion of the trial denture is checked along with the required freeway space. Once the patient is satisfied with the esthetics of the trial denture, the clinician can proceed toward the definitive impression stage.

## Final Impression Procedure

Areas of overextension are reduced to create adequate space to allow for the thickness of the impression material. If under extended, then the peripheral extensions are to be corrected by adding materials like greens stick compound before making the final impressions. Here, closed mouth technique is recommended.

### Step by Step Impression Making Procedure

- Remove gross undercuts and correct the under extended borders if needed
- Spread the selected final impression material in the maxillary replica and seat it with an upward pressure until its fully seated
- The border molding procedures are done to get the correct extensions and then the mandibular replica is placed in the mouth and the patient is asked to close gently in centric
- The final manipulation of the tissues is done with the mouth closed
- Once set the replicas are removed and the maxillary impression checked
- Reseat the upper impression and place the final impression material filled mandibular replica in the mouth
- Once the tongue movements are accomplished, the patient is directed to close the mouth gently so that the teeth touch evenly
- The final manipulation for the mandibular impression is also done with the mouth closed
- On setting, remove the replicas and check for discrepancies if any
- The technician takes over the replicas for flasking, packing and denture finishing to be delivered to the clinician.

## ■ MODIFIED DUPLICATION TECHNIQUE

**Purpose:** Duplicating prosthesis incorporating significant changes or corrections in the duplicated dentures.

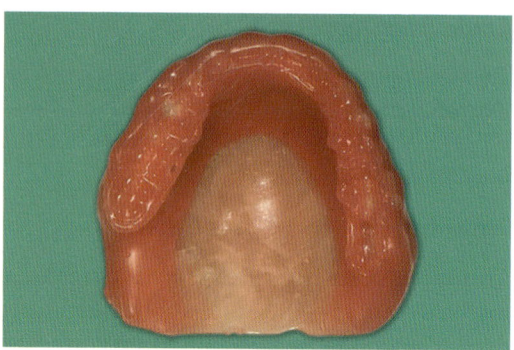

Fig. 10.4.15: Incremental addition of wax to the occlusal surface until the correct Vertical dimension and acceptable occlusion is achieved

In this technique, apart from copying the shape of polished surface many corrections such as occlusal surface changes can also be made. Once the replicas are produced utilizing the above method, wax is incrementally added to the occlusal surface of the replicas until perfect contact is achieved at the enhanced vertical dimension **(Fig. 10.4.15)**. Freeway space is checked and the replicas are sealed at the new vertical. After shade selection, the sealed replicas are sent to the laboratory for the needful as described in the previous section.

## ACRYLIC TEMPLATE TECHNIQUE FOR DENTURE DUPLICATION

**Purpose:** Replicate tooth position and shape of the polished surface.

### Step by Step Procedure

- Laboratory silicon is used to make impressions of old dentures and clear acrylic replicas are made
- Rigidity of the heavy body silicon is enough to be used without additional support and is an advantage in comparison to alginate which slumps. However, for support and extra rigidity it is imperative that two metal stock trays be used for individual dentures
- These clear acrylic replicas are tried in the mouth and checked for discrepancies
- Undercuts are removed if required and the acrylic replicas are used as custom trays for impression making

- A definitive impression is made for maxillary and mandibular arch with ZOE impression paste or light body silicon using an open mouth technique. The material used for wash impression must be fluid enough to ensure minimal increase in vertical dimension
- It is advisable to make vents in the palatal zone of the replica prior to making the final impressions to eliminate pressure build up. These relief holes also help in achieving thin impressions keeping the increase in vertical dimension to a minimum.
- The replicas serve as custom trays and bite blocks
- Jaw relation is recorded with the help of aluwax or bite registration material at the same visit eliminating the need for an added appointment
- In the laboratory, the acrylic is trimmed and the teeth are placed in the desired position. A putty index helps in copying the position of the teeth
- Once the try-in is approved by the patient, the denture is sent for acrylization.

The term copying here is synonymous to duplicating or replicating some features of the old dentures. There are three surfaces to a denture:

1. Occlusal: The tooth surface
2. Intaglio: The impression surface
3. Cameo: The polished surface.

The used dentures should ideally be examined carefully to decide which surface needs to be duplicated. Once decided, any of the above mentioned techniques with modifications can be used.

The main advantages of duplicating a denture with these techniques are improved patient acceptance for the prosthesis and fewer appointments leading to reduced treatment time.

## PROBLEMS WITH COMPLETE DENTURE DUPLICATION

Denture duplication currently is not commonly used in daily practice. This is due to subpar fabrication after using duplication techniques as experienced by many clinicians. The inability to diagnose faults in the old prosthesis prior to the fabrication of a duplicate denture plays a major role in failures.

## Drawbacks

- Inability to diagnose technically inadequate dentures
- Increased vertical dimension
- Compromised occlusion
- Overextended dentures
- Inability to record correct post dam
- Flabby/compromised tissues may lead to unstable dentures.

Commonly, patients present the clinician with an unacceptable old worn denture and request a replica as they have become accustomed to the denture with time. Dentists should be careful to replicate such dentures which are technically incorrect. These dentures should not be considered for replication in entirety. The dentist must diagnose the problems such as attrition, reduced vertical dimension and others using the replicas for trial modifications which can be later finalized without altering the old denture. It is effective only if the clinician understands the limitations of replicating dentures.

## Conclusion

- This technique has its share of drawbacks as many times the old denture to be replicated is not in best of conditions. Therefore, the clinician has to be very careful in choosing patients for copy dentures.
- Preserving and replicating the shape of polished surfaces of old dentures may help the patient in adapting to the new ones with ease.

# Clinical Cases

| | | |
|---|---|---|
| Case 1 | Complete Dentures for Compromised Ridges | 235 |
| Case 2 | Immediate Dentures with Chairside Soft Reline | 237 |
| Case 3 | Denture Fabrication with Modified Neutral Zone Technique | 241 |
| Case 4 | Immediate Dentures | 245 |

*We all begin our life's journey without them, let's not end the same way*

Shivangi

# Case 1

# Complete Dentures for Compromised Ridges

A 65 years old edentulous patient presented with compromised maxillary and mandibular ridges. After a thorough examination, it was decided to use conventional impression technique for the maxillary arch and "All green technique, modification of McCord's technique" for the mandibular arch. During the try in stage a wax cheek plumper was also introduced to improve buccal fullness, which was maintained in the final denture to enhance facial esthetics.

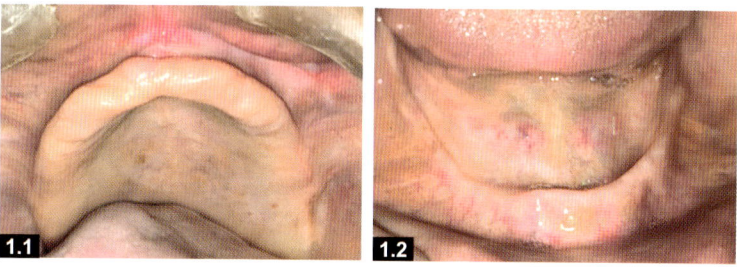

**Fig. 1.1:** Maxillary edentulous arch. **Fig 1.2:** Mandibular resorbed edentulous arch

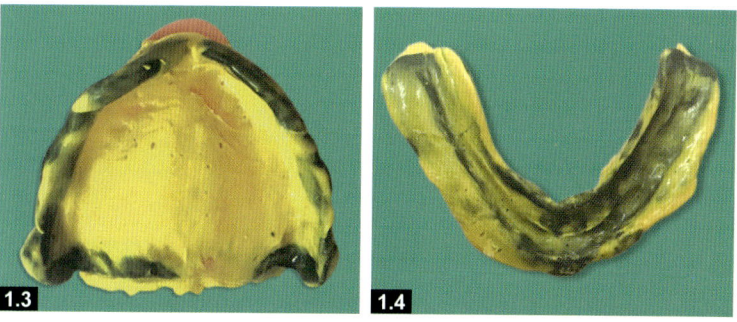

**Fig. 1.3:** Conventional maxillary final impression. **Fig 1.4:** Mandibular secondary impression utilizing all green tecnique for recording a severly resorbed ridge

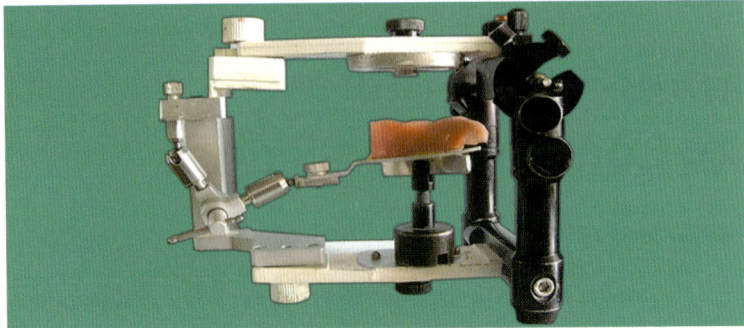

Fig. 1.5: Orientation relation transferred with the help of a facebow to a semi adjustable articulator

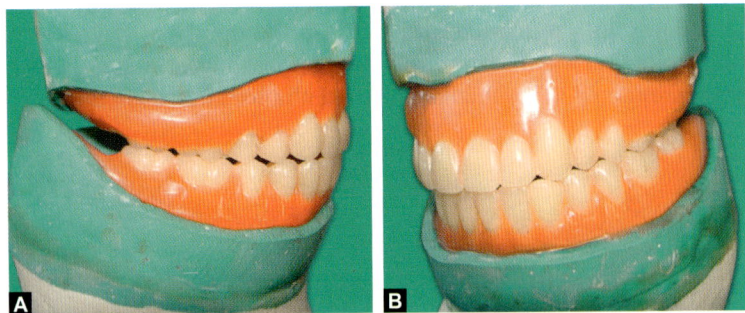

Figs 1.6A and B: Try In Stage: Balanced wax up denture with cheek plumper to compensate for buccal fullness (A) Right and (B) Left lateral view

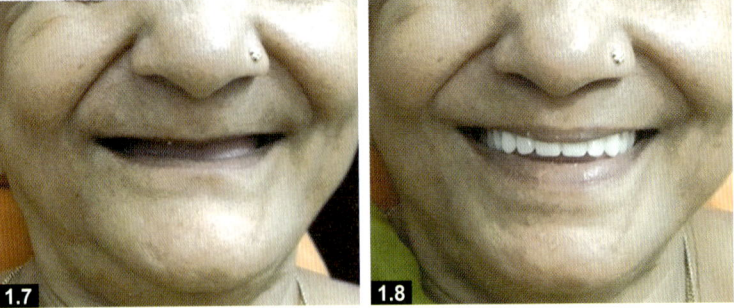

Fig. 1.7: Pre treatment picture without dentures. Fig 1.8: Post treatment picture with dentures

# Case 2

# Immediate Dentures with Chairside Soft Reline

A 68 years old, female patient suffered from bells palsy. On intra oral examination, there were 6 periodontally compromised maxillary anterior teeth and 3 root stumps in the mandible were present. After explaining the patient about various treatment modalities, she chose to go ahead with Immediate Complete Dentures.

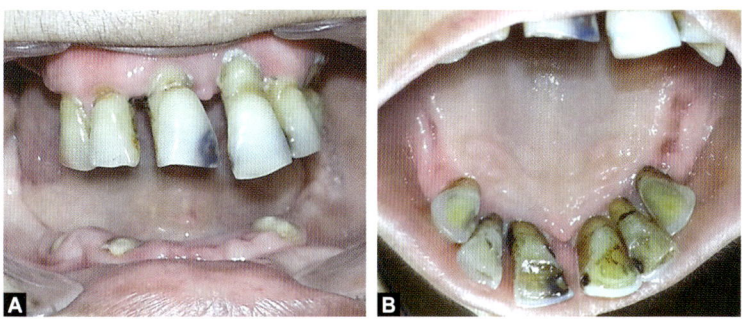

**Figs 2.1A and B:** Initial situation

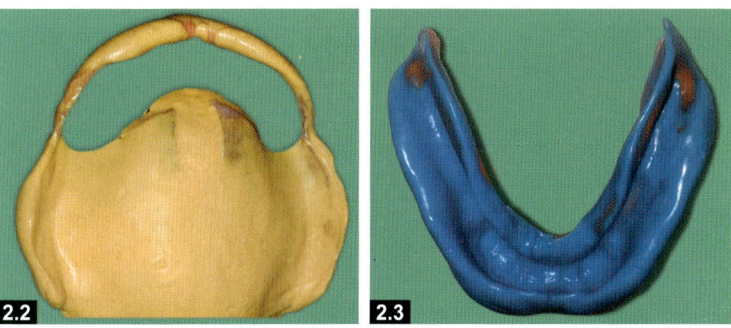

**Fig 2.2:** Two stage final impression technique-maxillary. **Fig 2.3:** Single stage final impression technique-mandibular

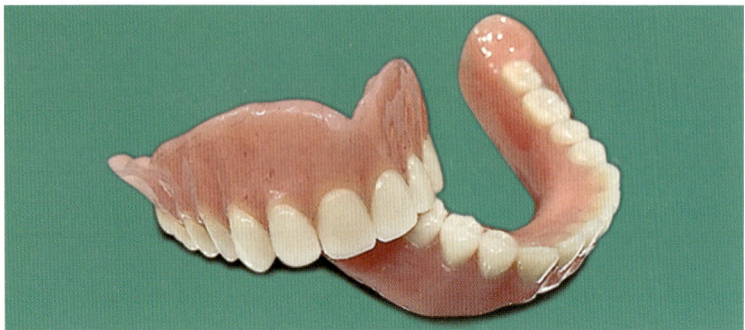

**Fig 2.4:** Final denture fabrication

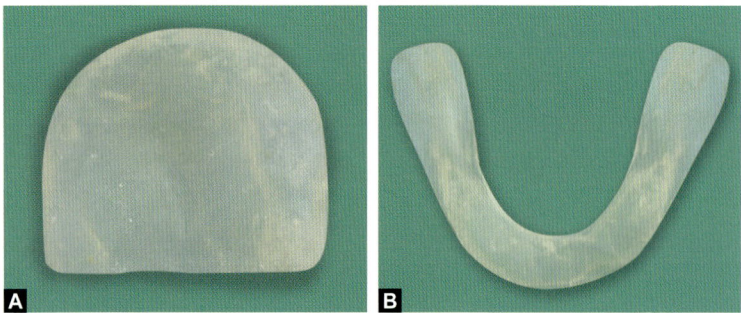

**Figs 2.5A and B:** Surgical template fabrication; (A) Maxillary. (B) Mandibular

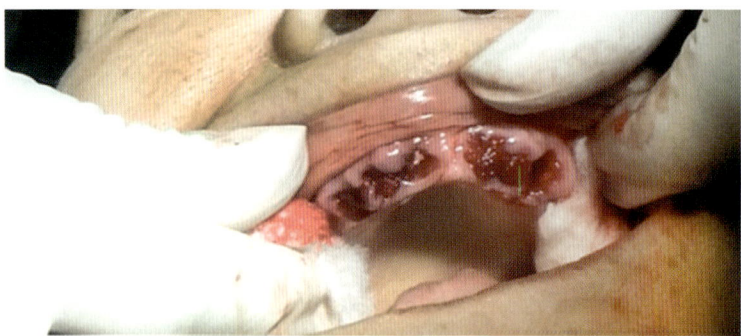

**Fig 2.6:** Extractions

## Case 2  Immediate Dentures with Chairside Soft Reline

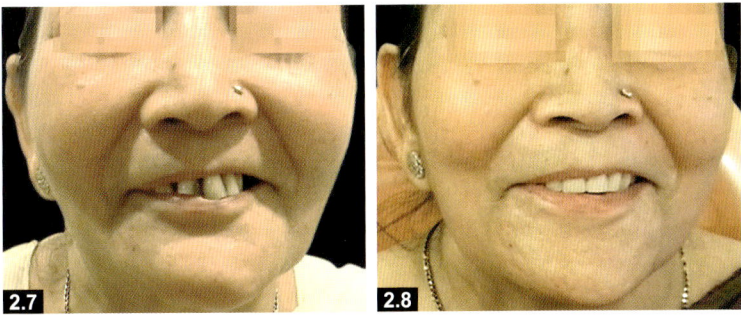

Fig 2.7: Preoperative frontal view of the patient.  Fig 2.8: Postoperative frontal view of the patient

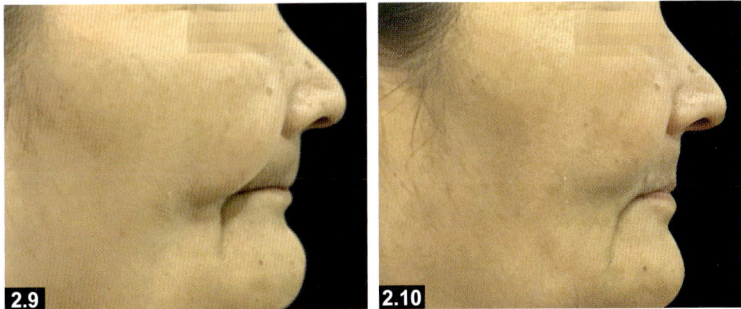

Fig 2.9: Preoperative profile view of the patient.  Fig 2.10: Postoperative profile view of the patient

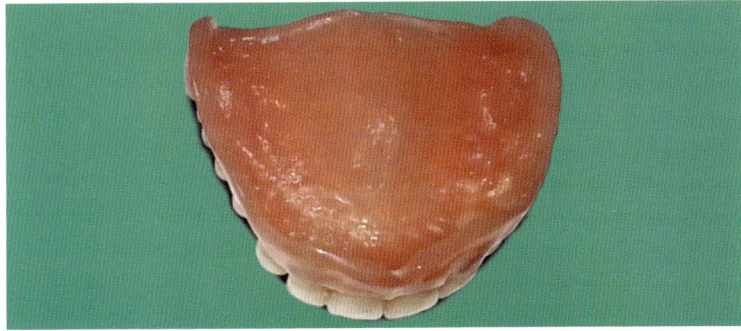

Fig 2.11: Chairside reline (Sofreline Tough) after two months to improve retention

# Case 3

# Denture Fabrication with Modified Neutral Zone Technique

An 82 years old female patient presented with partially edentulous maxillary and mandibular arches resulting in imbalance of circumoral muscles, leading to complete esthetic failure. The mandibular ridge showed 3 periodontally compromised teeth with Grade III mobility. After initial extraction of those 3 teeth, the ridge became highly uneven. Recent extractions led to discrepancy in alveolar bone thickness and levels showing extreme resorption in all other areas of the ridge. Patient already had a maxillary interim partial denture and desired a complete mandibular denture to match the upper. Patient was a cancer survivor and had undergone tracheostomy last year. Taking patient's age, medical condition into consideration, bone levels and desire for a removable denture, certain specific modifications were planned. Modified McCord's technique for final impression, modified neutral zone for the mandible with functional impression material to record the precise placement of teeth and tongue space were used. Eventually, chairside soft reline was accomplished with satisfactory results.

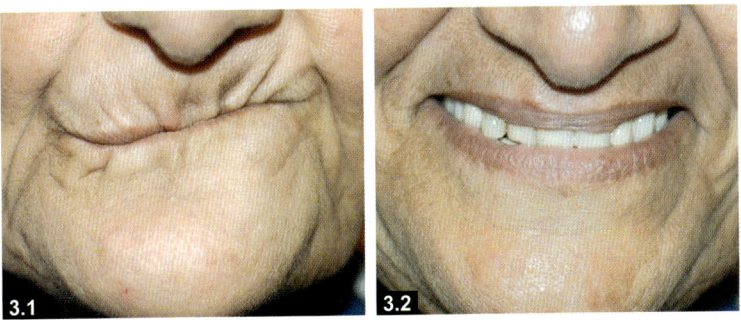

**Fig. 3.1:** Prior to placement of dentures. **Fig 3.2:** Post denture insertion

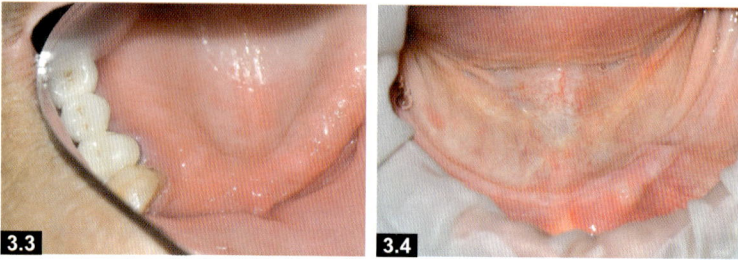

**Fig 3.3:** Partially edentulous maxilla. **Fig 3.4:** Unevenly resorbed mandibular ridge post extractions

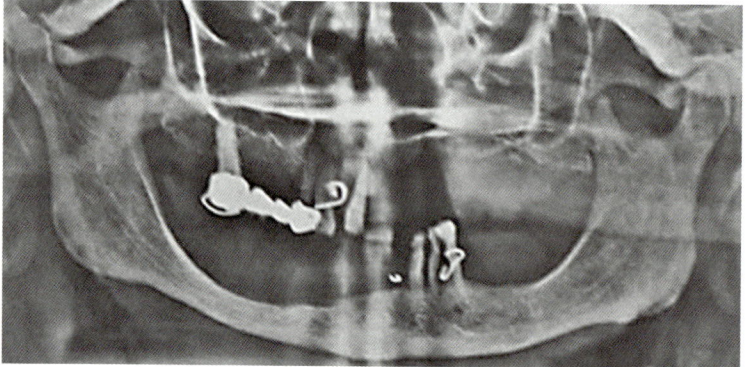

**Fig 3.5:** Orthopantomogram: Grade III mobile lower teeth visible. These 3 teeth were extracted prior to denture fabrication

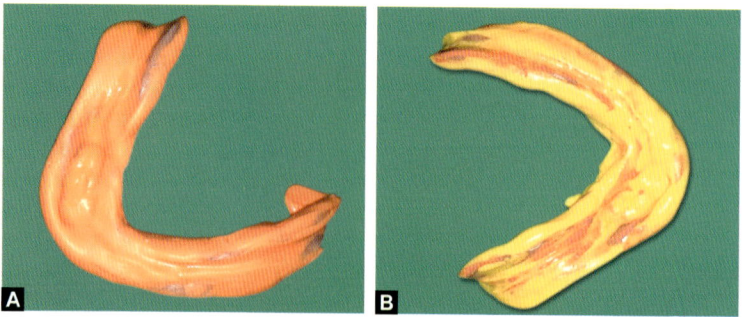

**Figs 3.6A and B:** Modified McCord's technique of recording final impression

## Case 3  Denture Fabrication with Modified Neutral Zone Technique

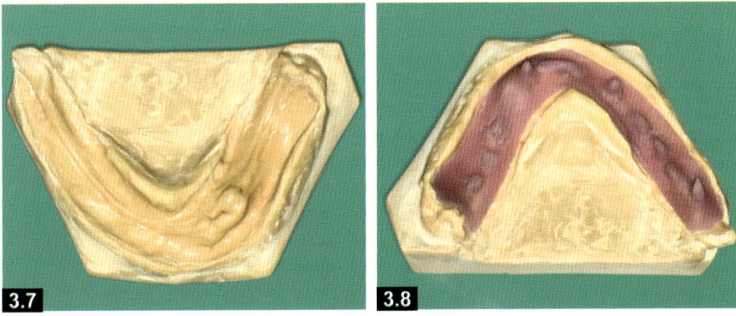

**Fig 3.7:** Final cast.  **Fig 3.8:** Denture base with retentive slots to support functional impression material

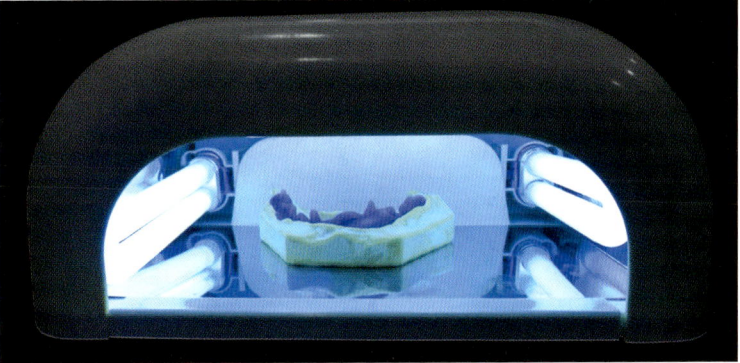

**Fig 3.9:** Light cure set of the denture base in a light cure (UV) box

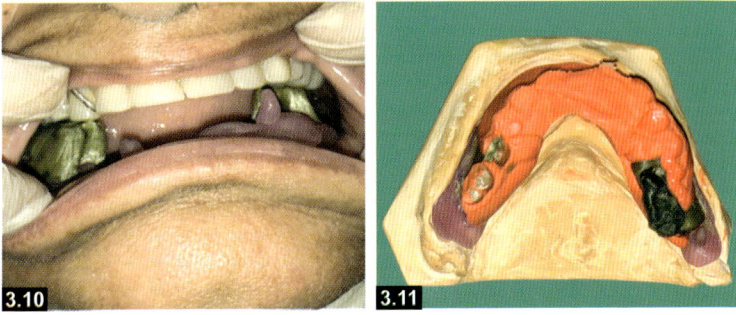

**Fig 3.10:** Aluwax centric stops created (For VD and Centric).  **Fig 3.11:** Modified neutral zone to achieve: tooth positioning, alveolo lingual sulcus and tongue space

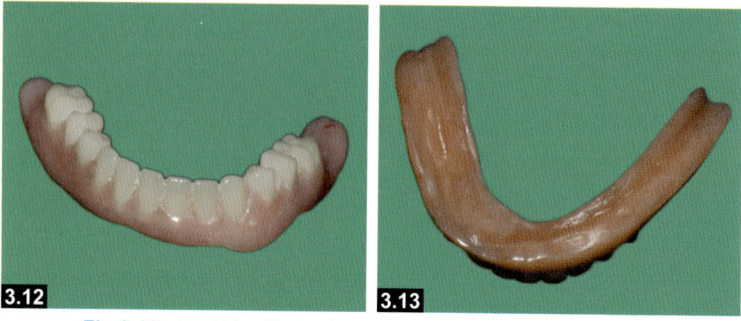

Fig 3.12: Final Mandibular denture.  Fig 3.13: Impression surface

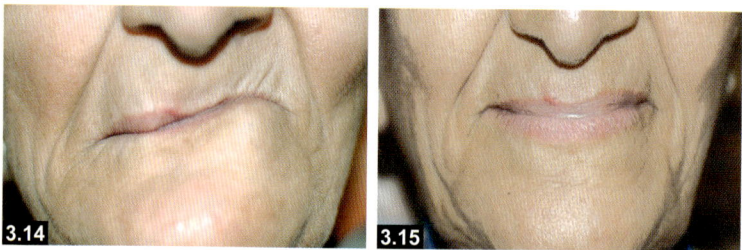

Fig 3.14: Pre operative picture without denture insertion.  Fig 3.15: Post operative picture with denture insertion

# Case 4

# Immediate Dentures

A 69 years old female patient presented with few remaining periodontally compromised teeth in both the arches. After detailing the patient about all treatments available, it was decided to go ahead with Immediate dentures. All the steps were diligently followed to ensure best results.

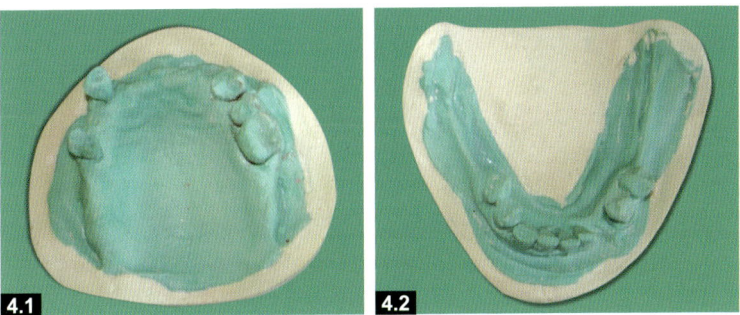

**Figs 4.1 and 4.2:** Maxillary and mandibular edentulous casts to showcase the remaining natural teeth

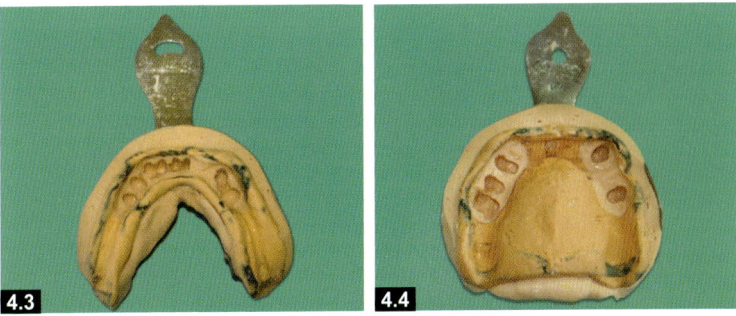

**Figs 4.3 and 4.4:** Two stage impression technique: First custom tray to record edentulous area and the second stock tray to record the teeth and to pick up the first tray

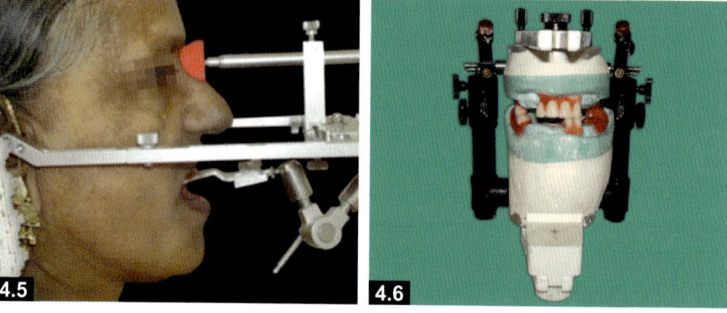

**Fig. 4.5:** Facebow record: Orientation relation. **Fig. 4.6:** Trimming of the stone teeth post try in for final denture fabrication

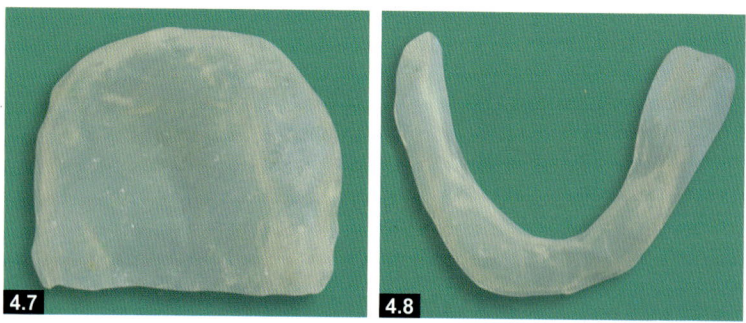

**Figs 4.7 and 4.8:** Maxillary and mandibular surgical splint to ensure stable denture base

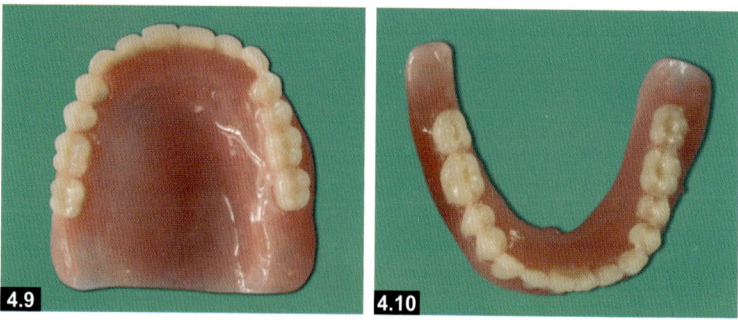

**Figs 4.9 and 4.10:** Final complete dentures for maxillary and mandibular arches

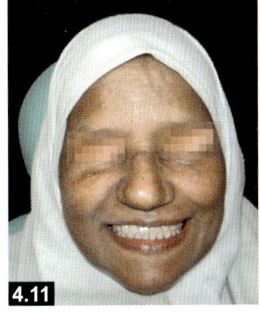 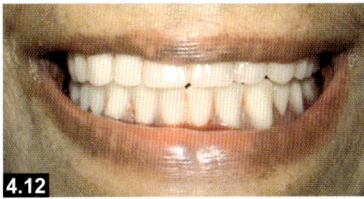

Fig. 4.11: Postoperative facial view of the patient. Fig. 4.12: Intra-oral picture after insertion of immediate denture

# Annexure

1. An alternative impression technique for complete dentures, Burak Yilmaz, February 2014 Volume 111, Issue 2, Pages 166-168 The journal of Prosthetic dentistry.
2. Complete dentures from planning to problem solving, Finbarr etal, Quentessentials of dental practice-12, Prosthodontics-2.
3. H A Young, September 1954 Volume 4, Issue 5, Pages 585-595 Objectives of complete denture treatments, The journal of Prosthetic dentistry.
4. *British Dental Journal* 188, 373 - 374 (2000). Published online: 8 April 2000 | doi:10.1038/sj.bdj.4800484. Complete dentures: an introduction, J F McCord[1] & A A Grant 2.
5. Winkler S. Symposium on Complete Dentures. *Dent Clin N Am* 1977; 21: 197-198.
6. McCord J F, Grant A A, Quayle A A. Treatment options for the edentulous mandible. Eur J Prosthodont Rest Dent 1992; 1: 19-23.
7. Complete denture copy technique—A practical application, Steven Soo, Singapore Dental Journal, Volume 35, December 2014, Pages 65-70.
8. G. E. Carlsson, "Clinical morbidity and sequelae of treatment with complete dentures," Journal of Prosthetic Dentistry, vol. 79, no. 1, pp. 17-23, 1998.
9. C. C. Wyatt, "The effect of prosthodontic treatment on alveolar bone loss: a review of the literature," The Journal of Prosthetic Dentistry, vol. 80, no. 3, pp. 362-366, 1998.
10. S. Winkler, Essentials of Complete Denture Prosthodontics, AITBS, New Delhi, India, 2nd edition, 2009.

11. G. Praveen, S. Gupta, S. Agarwal, and S. K. Agarwal, "Cocktail impression technique: a new approach to atwood's order vi mandibular ridge deformity," Journal of Indian Prosthodontist Society, vol. 11, no. 1, pp. 32–35, 2011.
12. R. M. Morrow, K. D. Rudd, and J. E. Rhoads, Dental Laboratory Procedures-Complete Dentures, vol. 1, Mosby, St. Louis, Mo, USA, 2nd edition, 1986.
13. A. Z. Zarb, C. L. Bolender, J. C. Hickey, and G. E. Carlsson, Boucher's Prosthodontic Treatment for Edentulous Patients, Elsevier Saunders, St. Louis, Mo, USA, 10th edition, 1990.
14. H. K. Tan, P. M. Hooper, and C. G. Baergen, "Variability in the shape of maxillary vestibular impressions recorded with modeling plastic and a polyether impression material," The International Journal of Prosthodontics, vol. 9, no. 3, pp. 282–289, 1996.
15. E. M. Applebaum and R. V. Mehra, "Clinical evaluation of polyvinylsiloxane for complete denture impressions," The Journal of Prosthetic Dentistry, vol. 52, no. 4, pp. 537–539, 1984.
16. J. F. McCord and K. W. Tyson, "A conservative prosthodontic option for the treatment of edentulous patients with atrophic (flat) mandibular ridges," British Dental Journal, vol. 182, no. 12, pp. 469–472, 1997.
17. The influence of clinical variables on patients' satisfaction with complete dentures, Marinus A.J. van Waas, The Journal of Prosthetic Dentistry, Volume 63, Issue 3, March 1990, Pages 307-310.
18. A comparison of lingualized occlusion and monoplane occlusion in complete dentures, Harold E Clough et al. The Journal of Prosthetic Dentistry, Volume 50, Issue 2, August 1983, Pages 176–179.
19. The neutral zone in complete dentures, Victor E. Beresin, The Journal of Prosthetic Denzistry, Volume 36, Issue 4, October 1976, Pages 356-367.
20. Factors influencing satisfaction with complete dentures in geriatric patients, A. Langer et al. The Journal of Prosthetic Dentistry, Volume 11, Issue 6, November–December 1961, Pages 1019–1031.
21. The retention of complete dentures, G.A. Lammie, JADA, October 1957 Volume 55, Issue 4, Pages 502–508.
22. Evidence-based guidelines for the care and maintenance of complete dentures, JADA, February 2011 Volume 142, Supplement 1, Pages 1S–20S.

23. Atwood DA. The reduction or residual ridges: a major oral disease entity. J Prosthet Dent 1971;26:266-278.
24. Heartwell CM, Rahn AO. Syllabus of complete dentures. 4th ed. Philadelphia: Lea & Febiger; 1986.
25. Sharry JJ (1974) Complete Denture Prosthodontics (3rdedn) Blakiston, New York, pp. 191-210.
26. Halperin G, Rogoff P (1988) Mastering the Art of Complete Dentures. Chicago, IL: Quintessence, pp. 43-51.
27. Smith PW, Richmond R, McCord JF (1999) The design and use of special trays in prosthodontics: guidelines to improve clinical effectiveness. Br Dent J 187: 423-426.
28. Christensen GJ (2008) Will digital impressions eliminate the current problems with conventional impressions? J Am Dent Assoc 139: 761-763.
29. Devlin H, Cash AJ, Watts DC (1995) Mechanical behaviour and structure of light-cured special tray materials. J Dent 23: 255-259.
30. Sheldon W (1996) Essentials of Complete Denture Prothodontics, 2nd ed. Philadelphia, PA: Ishiyaku Euro America, pp. 88-106.
31. Zarb GA, Bolender CL, Carlsson GE (1999) Boucher's Prosthodontic Treatment for Edentulous Patients (11thedn) St. Louis, MO: Mosby, pp. 3123-3123.
32. Shetty S, Nag PVR, Shenoy KK (2007) A review of the techniques and presentation of an alternate custom tray design. JIPS 7: 8-11.
33. Zinner ID, Sherman H (1981) An analysis of the development of complete denture impression techniques. J Prosthet Dent 46: 242-249.
34. Immediate denture construction: The impression phase, James R Lambrecht, The journal of prosthetic dentistry, March 1968Volume 19, Issue 3, Pages 237–245.
35. Immediate denture fabrication: a clinical report, Sergio Caputi, Ann Stomatol (Roma). 2013 Jul-Sep; 4(3-4): 273–277.
36. Zarb GA, Bolender CL. Prosthodontic treatment for edentulous patients. 12th Ed. Vol. 8. St. Louis: The C.V. Mosby Co; 2004. pp. 123–159.
37. Seals RR, Kuebker WA, Stewart KI. Immediate complete dentures. Dent Clin North Am. 1996;40:151–167.
38. Soni A. Trial anterior artificial tooth arrangement for an immediate denture patient: a clinical report. J Prosthet Dent. 2000;84:260–3.

39. Fractured Denture Repairs, Mark H. Johnson, May 1982 Volume 104, Issue 5, Pages 644–645.
40. Hummel SK, et al. Quality of removable partial dentures worn by the adult U.S. population. J Prosthet Dent. 2002 Jul;88(1):37-43.
41. N Z Dent J. 1992 Apr;88(392):56-9, The copy denture technique, Treasure P.

# Index

Page numbers followed by *f* refer to figure, *fc* refer to flow chart and *t* refer to table.

## A

Abrasion, signs of excess  16*f*
Acid abrasion  16*f*
Acrylic denture teeth, attrited  131*f*
Acrylic resin  88
Acrylic teeth  228*f*
Acrylic template technique  230
Adhesive  170
    powder  170*f*
Adhesive-error relationship  170*f*
Alveolar bone  3
Alveolar resorption, gross  11*f*
Alveolar ridge resorption  5*f*
Alveolo lingual sulcus  243*f*
Analgesic ointments  172
Angular chelitis  28*f*, 152*f*
Arch form  109
    types of  111*f*
Arcon articulator  124*f*
Atwoods classification  8, 8*f*

## B

Bard-Parker blade  206
Beading  82

Bone
    reduction  29
    resorption, severe  167
British Dental Association's Infection  61
Buccal aspect  3
Buccal corridor  114, 115*f*
    factors affecting  115
Buccal freni  50
Buccal mucosa  35*f*

## C

Calcium deficiency  39, 39*f*
    treatment  39
Candida albicans  34
Candidiasis  34, 152, 167
    aetiology of  34*f*
Canine prominence  115
Cast
    final  243*f*
    mandibular primary  183*f*
    maxillary primary  183*f*
Cephalometric radiograph, lateral  15
Chairside reline  239*f*

Cheek extended
  downward 77f
  inward 77f
  outward 77f
Chewing center located brain stem 162f
Chromatic alginate 52f
Circumoral musculature 165f
Clinical impression procedures 205
Cold cure acrylic custom trays 73f
Complete alveolingual sulcus 80f
Condylar disc assembly inset 4f
Condylar guidance 124f
Condyle disk assembly 87f
Conventional hand mixing technique 52
Cuspal inclination 125f
Custom tray fabrication 70

# D

Dawson's bimanual manipulation 101
Dental plaster base 63f
Dentition, patients with terminal 28
Dentogenic concept 106
Denture 142f, 225f
  aches with new 166
  adhesive application, procedure for 170
  base
    area 122f
    characterization 115, 116f
    classification 90t
    in light cure box 243f
    in wax 116f
    material, colors of 116f
    strengtheners 216
    with retentive slots 243f
  bearing area
    inflamed 201f
    mandibular 47f
  bearing tissues 36
  changed with new 164
  complete 49, 138, 165f, 199, 235
  concept of new 162
  copy 219, 221
  dirty 17f
  duplication 230
    complete 231
  esthetics 105
  examination
    of old 4
    existing old 16
  existing 224f
  fabricated complete 202f
  fabrication 99, 241
    complete 15f
    final 238f, 246f
  facial 28f
  final mandibular 244f
  for mandibular arches, complete 246f
  for maxillary arches, complete 246f
  fracture 211, 214
    types of 211
  hygiene 168
  hyperplasia 201f
  immediate 179, 181, 237, 245
    complete 237
  impression procedures for 43
  in place 6f
  influence of complete 5f
  insertion 139, 141
    after extractions 193f
    post-operative with 244f
    pre-operative without 244f
  light cured 89f
  maintenance with patient education 159, 161
  mandibular 37f, 145f, 148f, 221f
    areas 146
    complete 8f
  mastication with new 162

maxillary 145*f*, 191*f*, 221*f*
   areas 145
      bearing areas 47*f*
midline fracture of mandibular 212*f*
new 222*f*
occlusion, complete 121
old 222*f*
oral feelings with new 163*f*
pains with new 166
palatal aspect of maxillary 16*f*
parts 214*f*
pieces, mismatched 16*f*
placement of 241*f*
post-treatment with 236*f*
preparation 204, 204*t*
pre-treatment without 236*f*
prosthesis
   advantages of 194
   disadvantage of 195
   complete 14, 37*f*, 130
relined maxillary 147*f*
repair 209, 211, 213*f*
   procedure, basic 213
   types of 212
replica, mandibular 227*f*
requirement 141*f*
retention 149
self repaired 171*f*
sore spot 18*f*
stage 229
   laboratory trial 228
stained mandibular 17*f*
stains on 169*f*
technique, copy 221, 223
teeth
   abnormal tear of 17*f*
   abnormal wear of 17*f*
   ortholingual 129*f*
   placement 190
trial 227
unclean 17*f*
unretentive 69
wear 27, 34, 199*f*, 200*f*
demonstrating, old 10*f*
first time 29
night time 169*f*
previous 33
with cheek plumper 236*f*
with putty impression 223*f*
Disinfection 60
Disto-buccal flange 145
Double metal tray technique 224, 225*f*, 226*f*
Double tray technique 184, 185*f*
Dynesthetic concept 106
Dysfunctional impression 59, 60*f*

# E

Edentulous
   arch, maxillary 235*f*
   maxilla, partially 242*f*
   maxillary arch 50*f*
   patient 10*f*
   patient without dentures 165*f*
Elastomeric silicon impressions 82
Epulis fissuratum 167
Esthetic 69
   dental proportion 115*f*
   evaluation 150

# F

Facebow 188*f*
   record 246*f*
Facial
   esthetics 235
   form 10
   frontal form 109
   line angles 20
   muscle tone 115
   profile 20, 109
      examination of 112*f*
   tissue, loss of 201*f*

Fracture
    of old mandibular complete denture 16*f*
    pieces 213*f*
    tooth repair 216
Frenum 20
Functional impression technique 206
Fungal infections 167

## G

Gingival characterization 117
Gingival margin 188
    bands 106
    level of 189*f*
Golden proportion 114
Gothic arch tracer 98, 100*f*

## H

Hanau's quint 124
Hard palate 11
Hard silicon 214*f*
Hard tissue 10
    procedures 29
    undercuts 12, 29
Health 36
Healthy oral tissues 47*f*
High frenum attachments 31
House mental classification 142
Hydrocolloid technique 53
Hygiene 168

## I

Impression procedure, final 229
Impression putty technique 225
Impression surface 244*f*
Impression technique
    final 74
    mandibular, final 237*f*
    maxillary, final 237*f*
Impression tray compound 53
In situ examination 18
Incisal display 7*f*, 7*t*

Incisal guidance, minimal 124*f*
Incisive papilla region 145
Incisors, wide central 108*f*
Inflamed tissues
    hypermobile 27*f*
    hyperplastic 203
Insertion timeline 192
Interarch space 109
Intercuspid distance 109
Interocclusal bite material 228*f*
Intraoral
    checks 145
    examination 4, 10
        complete 49

## K

Kennedy's class I, modification 185

## L

Labial freni 50
Labial frenum 13*f*, 58*f*
Labial undercut 186*f*
Laboratory communication 133, 135
Lesions 4
Lingual flange, anterior 80
Lingualized occlusion 129, 129*f*
Lip
    fullness 7, 91
    length 7, 7*f*, 7*t*, 91, 109
    support 6, 20
        partial 9
        reduced 5*f*
        ridge form on 9*t*
    thickness 109
    unsupported 9
Long face syndrome 95*f*, 151*f*

## M

Mandibular
    anterior ridge alveoplasty 30*f*
    arch 50*t*, 58, 105*f*, 121*f*

# Index

cast 71*f*
impression 56
jaw 39*f*
replicas 228*f*
residual ridge 11*f*
resorbed edentulous arch 235*f*
ridge 18*f*, 50*f*
    post extractions 242*f*
secondary impression 235*f*
sharp residual ridge 26*f*
tori 26*f*
tray border molding 79
wax rim 93, 93*f*
Massetric notch 175*f*
Maxilla
    clear acrylic template in 193*f*
    relations of 87
Maxillary
    anterior
        ridge 186*f*
        teeth 237
    arch 13*f*, 50*t*, 57, 115, 121*f*, 186*f*
    cast 71*f*
    custom tray border extension 70
    impression 56
    occlusal wax rim 91
    posterior teeth 115
    primary impression 58*f*
    replicas 228*f*
    teeth in wax, replicated 227*f*
    tray 80
        border molding 76
    wax rim 98*f*
        horse shoe shaped 91*f*
Maxillomandibular relations 85, 87, 187
McCord's technique 241, 242*f*
Mechanical machine mixing technique 53
Metal flask technique 225
Metal stock trays 55*f*
Monoplane occlusal scheme 128, 128*f*

Mouth technique
    closed 205
    open 205
Mouth, dryness of 38
Mucoceles 28, 35
Mucosa 4
Mucous membrane biotype 20
Muscle
    mass, reduction in 38
    of modiolus affect 70
    tone 6, 20, 195
Mylohyoid ridge 50

## N

Nasolabial angle 92, 92*f*
Nick and notch method 97
Niswonger's method 187
Nutrition 36

## O

Occlusal concepts 130
Occlusal equilibration 175*f*
Occlusal schemes 127
Occlusal wax rim fabrication 91
Occlusion, plane of 125
Oral
    candidiasis 35*f*
    cavity, preparation of 23, 25
    checks, extra 143
    examination, extra 4, 5
    hygiene 168
    lesions, examination of irreversible 14
    mucosa 13
    tissues 135
    tracers, extra 99*f*
Orthopantomogram 15, 36*f*, 39*f*

## P

Palates pose, deep 12*f*
Palatogram 155
Papillary hyperplasia 27*f*, 33

Peeling of soft line  207f
Permanent denture base  90
    fabrication of  91
Permanent soft reline materials  206
Plaster, place of  214f
Plastic disposable stock trays  55f
Polished surface  144
Polymorph beads  73f
Preprosthetic surgery  13
Pressure indicating paste  175f
Probable cause  19
Proclined maxillary anterior teeth  186f
Prominent chin  6f
Prosthesis, finishing of  190
Protein
    deficiency  39
        treatment  40

## R

Realeff effect  49
Reline kits  172
Relining procedures  197, 199
Residual alveolar ridge  20
    form  7
Residual ridge  50
Retention cyst  28
Retromolar pad area  50
Retromylohyoid arch  50
Ridge
    compromised  235
    relation  11, 109
Root carving  151f

## S

Saliva  14, 21
Salivary flow, excess  164
Silverman's closest speaking space  157
Single tray
    impression  184f
    technique  183f

Soap box technique  224
Sofreline tough  239f
Soft hypermobile tissues  33
Soft tissue  4, 13
    lesions  21, 34
Spacer wax placement  71f
Speech
    unfavorable  195
    with new dentures  166
Speech sound  157f
    evaluation  156t
    specific  156
Stock trays  54
    types of  54fc
Surgical template fabrication  189, 238f
    mandibular  238f
    maxillary  238f

## T

Taste sensation, lack of  38
Temporary denture bases  90
Temporomandibular joint  4f
    examination  5
Terminal dentition  26f
Tissue  204t
    adaptation to  147
    compromised  35
    conditioner  203f
        stages of  204t
    dehydration  38
        treatment  39
    hyperplastic  13f
    placement of  193f
    preparation  204
    preservation  167
    red inflamed  13f
    side/intaglio  143
    trauma
        hard  192f
        soft  192f
Tokuyama tough medium  37f

Tongue 14, 21, 38*f*
  space 243*f*
Tooth
  anatomy 129
    types of 123*fc*
  anterior 112*f*
  color 112
  form of 111
  fracture 211
    dislodged 171*f*
    multiple 211
    single 211, 212*f*
  loss of 5*f*
  molds 122
  natural 216
  occlusion, natural 121
  pale 108*f*
  placement 188
  positioning 243*f*
  removal 189*f*
  replacement of 181
  rounded 108*f*
  selection 111
  shape of 111
  size of 111
  slots for 226*f*
  small 108*f*
    portion of fractured 216*f*
  visibility 91
  wear 19
    cause of 19*t*

    wear, excessive 19
      anterior 19
      posterior 19
Tori 12, 20, 31, 31*fc*
Torus palatinus 182*f*

## V

Valsalva's maneuver 76
Vents in
  mandibular tray, placement of 81*f*
  maxillary tray, placement of 80*f*
Vents, purpose of 81
Vestibular sulci 50
Vitamin
  depletion 40
    treatment 40
  supplements 40

## W

Wax teeth 227*f*, 228*f*

## X

Xerostomia 167

## Z

Zinc oxide eugenol impression paste 74